MEDICINE IS THE BEST LAUGHTER™

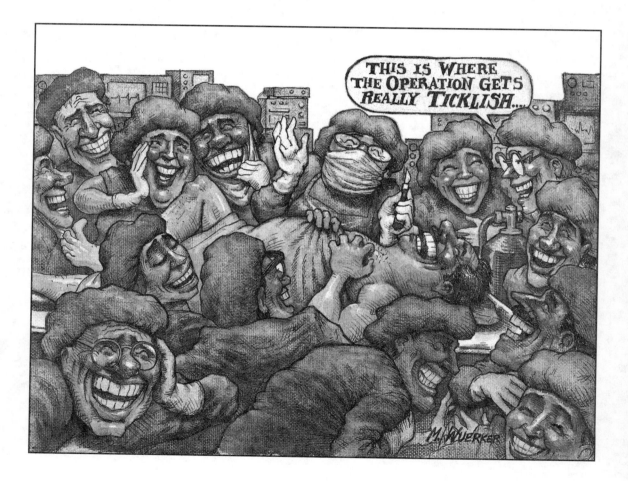

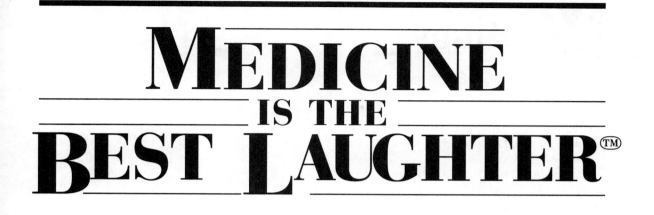

MEDICINE IS THE BEST LAUGHTER™

EDITED AND COMPILED

BY

GIDEON BOSKER, M.D.

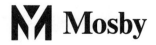 Mosby

St. Louis Baltimore Boston Carlsbad Chicago Naples New York Philadelphia Portland
London Madrid Mexico City Singapore Sydney Tokyo Toronto Wiesbaden

Mosby

Dedicated to Publishing Excellence

Publisher: Anne S. Patterson
Editor: Susie H. Baxter
Developmental Editor: Ellen Baker Geisel
Project Manager: Gayle May Morris
Production Manager: Mary Cusick Drone
Manufacturing Supervisor: Kathy Grone
Designer: Susan Lane

Cover art: Matt Wuerker

Printed in the United States of America
Composition by Top Graphics
Printing/binding by Plus Communications

Mosby-Year Book, Inc.
11839 Westline Industrial Drive
St. Louis, Missouri 64146

International Standard Book Number
0-8016-8113-8

95 96 97 98 / 9 8 7 6 5 4 3 2

To
my mother
DORKA BOSKER
who is both
chronologically gifted
and
very funny

Preface

According to an old saying, "Laughter Is The Best Medicine." But all these years of clipping medical cartoons, scribbling anecdotes, and scouring used book stores for classics of visual humor have taught me that *Medicine Is The Best Laughter*™.

I've been collecting medical cartoons for more than 15 years. I have hundreds and hundreds of them, culled from myriad sources, ranging from *The New Yorker, National Lampoon,* and *Saturday Evening Post* to *The National Enquirer,* archival collections, and the daily newspaper. They now fill every spare nook and cranny of every bookshelf and desk drawer. With friends, family, and colleagues sending me clippings from all over the world, these cartoons sometimes seem to breed before my very eyes. They are my *Comedy Club* without walls. And I confess that I sometimes read the gag lines aloud to myself, if for no other reason than to elevate the stature of these cartoons to that of living, breathing theater.

My medical cartoon collection has become my paper auditorium, packed with hundreds of comedians, cartoonists, and satirists, each letting me in on a private joke. The cartoons constantly fascinate me. They can distill the intricate agony and ecstasy–driven world of medicine into a simple formula that does what every healer should be able to do—make us smile.

That medical situations should put people *in stitches* should surprise no one. After all, the world of medicine contains all the necessary ingredients required to make people laugh. It is sometimes wonderful and sometimes sad; but often it is a whacky, whimsical, and entirely unpredictable sphere of human life that inspires infinite curiosity and a boundless appetite for laughter.

It is well accepted that encounters with physicians and nurses have the capacity for unmasking all of us at our most vulnerable moments. These delicate situations are the fuel for much of the humor we associate with the healing arts.

Visual humorists, in particular, have demonstrated an uncanny ability to capitalize on these situations. For example, it is no wonder that a cartoon in which a policeman attempts to control a curious mob on a busy street with the declaration, "All right, ALL RIGHT—I'm sure you've all seen somebody getting an enema before . . ." sends a tingle through our funny bone. And the patient who appears at his doctor's office requesting "one of those operations I heard about on *All Things Considered*" is yet another reminder of just how bizarre the world of medical information can be.

Because medicine also balances precariously on the delicate cusp between agony and ecstasy, between hope and tragedy, between loss and opportunity, it also is uniquely positioned for the kind of topsy-turvy reframings that cast critical situations into an absurd light and that, in the process, generate timeless examples of humor. Consider the following examples. The obstetrician-gynecologist consoles a despondent patient with the following note of reassurance: "You're not infertile, Mrs. Simmons. Perhaps you just don't breed well in captivity." Setting his characters in the post-op recovery suite, one medical humorist, Charles Rodrigues, weaves the following zany twist: "His stitches can come out in seven or eight days," confides a surgeon to his patient's wife, "and I see no reason why you can't begin denying him sex again in about two weeks." In the doctor's waiting room, this absurd perspective is pushed to its limits when a nurse informs her patient that, "The doctor will be out to see you as soon as he gets rid of those pesky guys from *60 Minutes.*"

Drugs can both cure diseases and cause potentially undesirable side effects; thus they have played a special role in the history of medicine and have inspired many medical cartoons. One of my favorites portrays a physician who, as he holds up a medication bottle with *two* pills, instructs a rather perplexed patient: "Take *one* upon going to bed, and the other *if* you wake up in the morning!" A medical researcher in a *Saturday Evening Post* cartoon raises the drug-related ante when he holds up a newly discovered medication and informs his superior, "Okay, so it doesn't cure anything, but the side effects are out of this world!" Even patients get into the act in the arena of pharmacologic humor. Sitting across from his date, a young man confides sheepishly, "Susan, I wish you'd had the chance to know me *before* my medication was adjusted."

Terror is to humor what coolness is to the neurosurgeon. Stated simply, it's the right stuff. In fact, the more terrifying a medical subject is, the more we like to see it exposed for the degree to which we have no control over it. And therefore we can't help but laugh at the cardiothoracic surgeon who, along with an assistant, presents himself at the bedside of his patient and declares, "I want to assure you the operation will go smoothly . . . I'll be assisted by Mr. Leonard, who took all my exams for me in medical school."

Terror as the flip side of comedy does not limit itself to corporeal humor. Lawyers, politicians, businessmen, and accountants also make cameo appearances in this comedy of errors. One *New Yorker* cartoon depicts a well-intentioned physician who reassures his patient by saying, "We medical practitioners do our very best, Mr. Nyman. Nothing is more sacred to us than the doctor-plaintiff relationship."

Freud claimed that both dreams and jokes reveal our inner truth, he also understood that the psychiatrist's couch is a hotbed for laughter. "Before I started therapy, I thought I was John F. Kennedy," complains a patient to his psychiatrist during his last session. "Now, I'm a nobody." In another cartoon, a therapist reassures his patient that he has "sufficient phobias, manias, and delusions to qualify for a handicap parking plate"; while in another, a psychiatrist urges his patient to "get out more, meet people, and make new enemies."

Although growing old is usually accompanied by bone wasting, it seems that the funny bone is spared. My mother at age 83 has been a lifelong inspiration to me as I gather anecdotes and cartoons that deal with the trials and tribulations of aging. "Thank You For Not Dying," reads a sign on the geriatric ward of a John Callahan cartoon, whereas in another panel by Steiner, the administrator at Shady Grove explains to a new resident, "We are a long-term care facility, Mrs. Williams, which means that over the long term you will get some care."

For years, I have been using cartoons in lectures that I have given to medical and nursing audiences around the country. What amazed me is how often my colleagues would approach me at the podium and say, "I enjoyed your lecture, Dr. Bosker . . . may I have a copy of some of your slides?" "Why, certainly," I would say, in the interest of advancing clinical medicine, "Which ones, in particular?" The inevitable reply, "The *cartoons.*"

I finally understood. For all of us in the healing arts, medical humor is a precious commodity. It is both a tension reliever and a safety valve. Although the primary purpose of this book is to provide entertainment and make us laugh, this extensive collection of cartoons and anecdotes can also be used to enhance medical presentations and lectures. Relieving audience tension by interspersing medical humor with scientific information is a proven and time-honored technique. To facilitate this process, the cartoons in *Medicine Is The Best Laughter*™ are organized according to medical specialties, themes, and categories so they can easily be matched with medical, nursing, and pharmacologic subjects.

Finally, there is no question that a sense of humor is a vital bodily function. A physician in one cartoon puts it nicely when he counsels his patient with this reassuring statement: "The human body is remarkably adaptive, Mr. Friar. Your other senses will compensate nicely for your lost sense of humor." Maybe, but maybe not. Still, it is very satisfying to know that if laughter, indeed, is so important to medicine, medicine itself can provide some of the best laughter around. And that's no joke.

GIDEON BOSKER

Acknowledgments

Completing this book required the collaboration and cooperation of many individuals and institutions. First of all, I thank all the actors in the drama, especially the cartoonists, artists, and humorists whose work has graced the pages of America's finest publications and has found its way into various libraries, collections, and archives throughout the country.

In this regard, special thanks go to cartoonists John Callahan, Peter Vey, Tom Cheney, Gahan Wilson, Libby Reid, Matt Groening, Charles Almon, John Piraro, Matt Jacobsen, Jim Unger, John McPherson, Bob Mankoff, Charles Rodrigues, Larry Trepel, Nick Downs, Gary Trudeau, Tom Wilson, Feggo, John Wise, Gary Larson, and the many other talented artists who were kind enough to permit publication of their work in this book. I extend a personal note of gratitude both to Lena Lencek, who painstakingly illustrated the anecdotes and provided consultation regarding cover design, and to Matt Wuerker, for his funny and beautiful cover illustration and design.

A book relying so heavily on visual material could not have come to fruition without the assistance of various libraries, newspaper syndicates, picture agencies, and individuals who were kind enough to supply and reproduce the visual material that appears herein. These individuals deserve special recognition for minimizing the usual tangle of red tape and byzantine regulations that impede archival research and for doing it with a smile. I stress that many of these curators and permissions directors were kind enough to rise above the call of duty and to actively participate in tracking down and collecting medical humor from their syndicates and newspaper archives. In this regard, I thank Mary C. Sugget, Permissions Director of Universal Press Syndicate, Liz Haberfeld (The Cartoon Bank, Inc.), Mary Beth Pacer (Tribune Media Services), Natasha Cooper (United Media), Sondra Robinson (Acme Features Syndicate), and Grace Darby *(The New Yorker)*.

Although the final selection of cartoons appearing in this book is the editor's responsibility, I am sincerely grateful to a number of devoted friends, interested loyalists, and colleagues who appeared on the scene and who, without solicitation, took the time to send clippings, relay humorous anecdotes, and offer their wise and impartial counsel regarding the final selection of cartoons for this project: Hollis Wilde, Paul and Susan Stander, J. Myron Berggren, David Wilson, Gayle Childers, Kent Anderson, Dorothy Bosker, Ellen Baker Geisel, Susie and Gil Baxter, Christy Steinhoff, Kirsten Pierce, Joanne Day, Richard and Leslie Day, Libby Reid, Bianca Lencek-Bosker, Lena Lencek.

I owe a special debt of gratitude to Kirsten Pierce, an extremely capable researcher, illustrator, and artist who was instrumental in tracking down a number of cartoonists, archival sources, and collections that appear in this book, for her superb organizational assistance during the home stretch of this project.

I acknowledge and express my sincere appreciation to the editorial team at Mosby. First, I am deeply grateful to George Parker, Vice President of Marketing, who had the vision, wisdom, and—perhaps, as important—a large enough funny bone to fuel his interest in the subject of medical humor. Mr. Parker, who was instrumental in setting the initial stage for Mosby's involvement in and commitment to this project, recognized the universal appeal of these cartoons. He, along with George Stamathis, former publisher at Mosby, and Anne Patterson, art-savvy Editor-in-Chief of Medical Books, green-lighted this unusual project. To them, I express my heartfelt thanks for permitting me to be involved with a book that has been such a pleasure to work on and that has given me so many laughs.

Finally, no project comes to completion without hands-on attention from a team of editors, designers, copy editors, and production coordinators. Stated simply, the Mosby team working on this project has been first class. In particular, I would like to thank Susan Lane and Mary Drone for making this book a feast for the eyes. And for their devotion, competence, professionalism, enthusiasm, and commitment to this project, I am grateful to Ellen Baker Geisel and Christy Steinhoff. Finally, for her encouragement, patience, wise guidance, and editorial panache, I would like to thank my editor, Susie Baxter, without whom this book would not be what it is.

GIDEON BOSKER

Contents

MEDICINE IS THE BEST LAUGHTER™

Bedside Manners

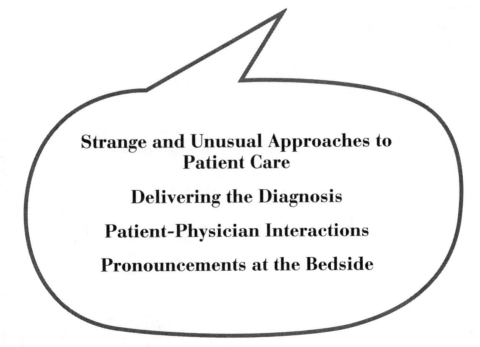

Strange and Unusual Approaches to
Patient Care

Delivering the Diagnosis

Patient-Physician Interactions

Pronouncements at the Bedside

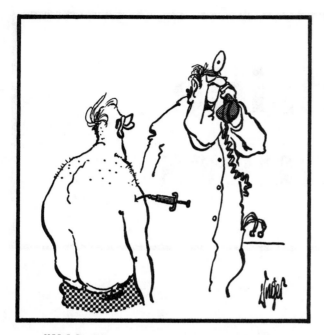

**"I'd better go now, Snookums.
I'm with a patient."**

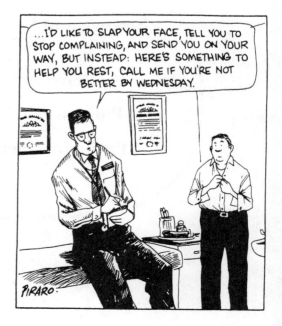

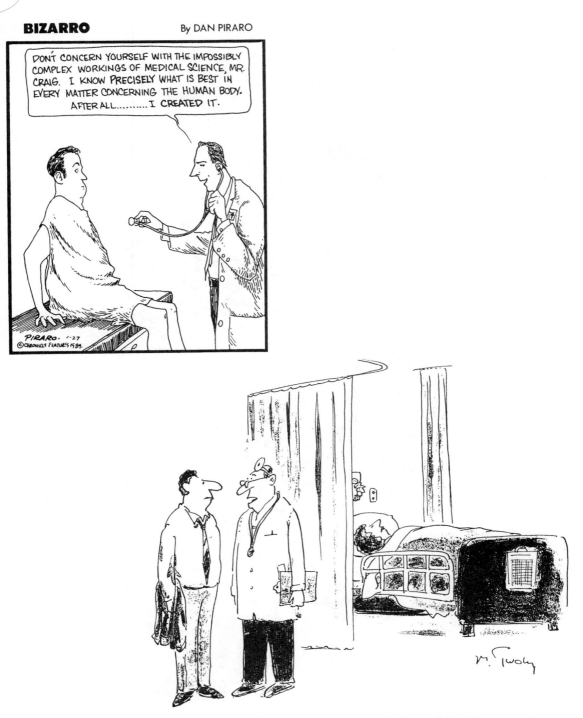

"It looks like she's going to have to be here for quite some time.
Do you need a loaner?"

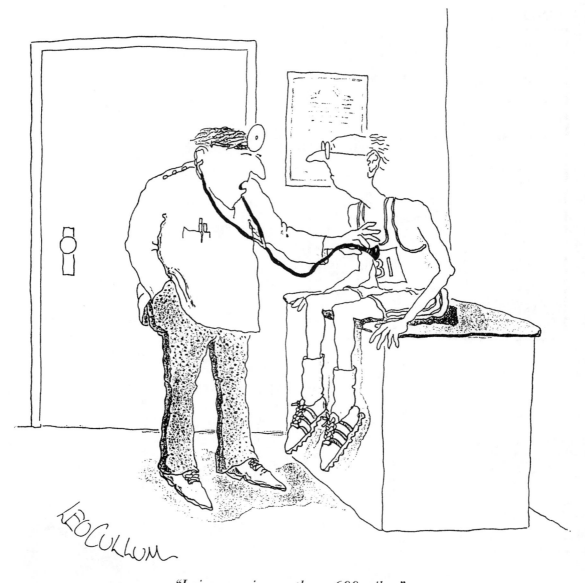

"I give you six months or 600 miles."

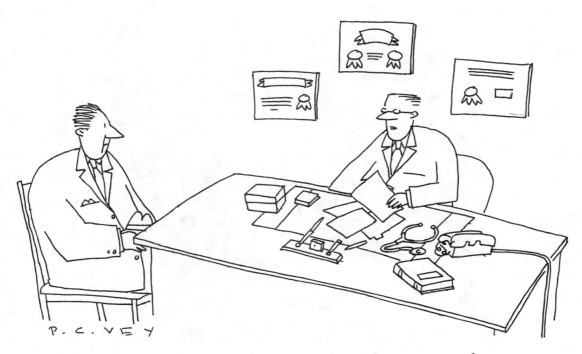

*"Frankly I see nothing wrong with you that a quarter of
a million dollars worth of medical care won't help."*

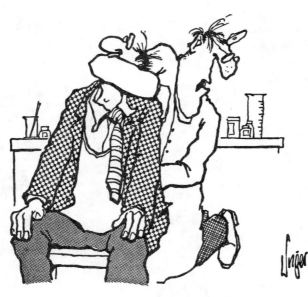

"Does that hurt?"

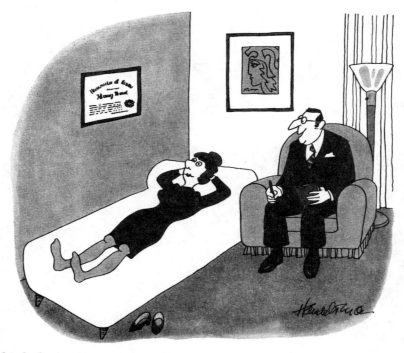

"I think that you are potentially a marvelous person. I think I am, too."

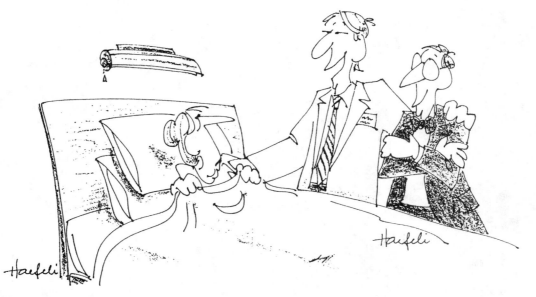

"I want to assure you the operation will go smoothly. I'll be assisted by Mr. Leonard who took all my exams for me in med school."

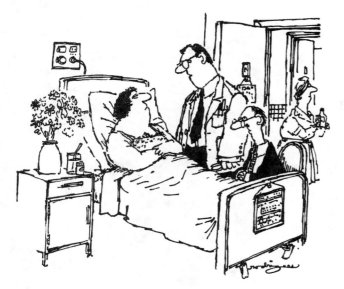

". . . the stitches can come out in 7 or 8 days
and I see no reason why you can't begin denying
him sex in about two weeks . . ."

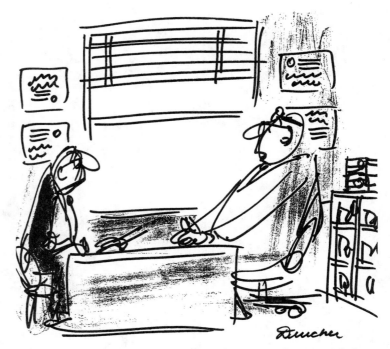

*"No wonder you're always sick. You make **me** sick."*

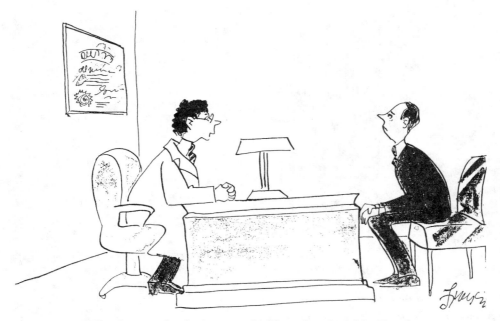

*"The human body is remarkably adaptive, Mr. Freelze.
Your other senses will compensate nicely for your
lost sense of humor."*

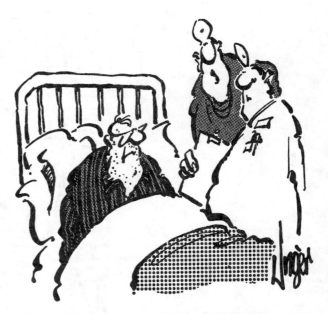

**"I explained the risks to his wife and
she thinks we should go for it."**

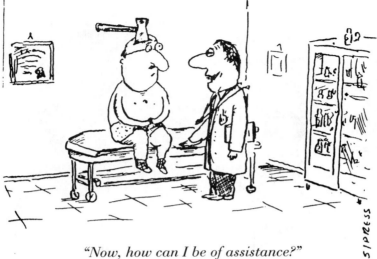

"Now, how can I be of assistance?"

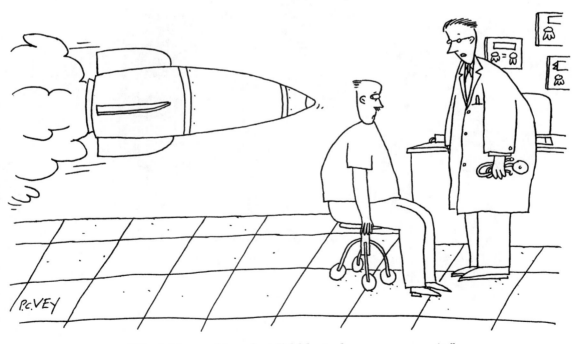

"Could be nothing, but I'd like to keep an eye on it."

9

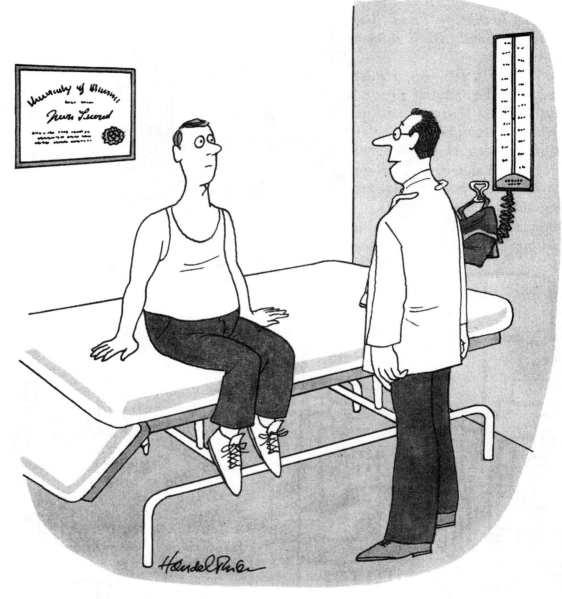

"*We medical practitioners do our very best, Mr. Nyman.
Nothing is more sacred to us than the doctor-plaintiff relationship.*"

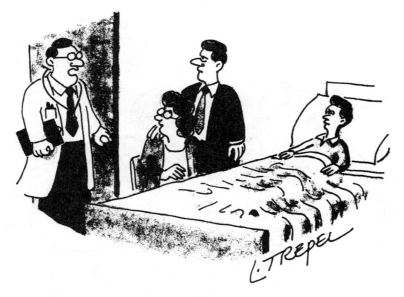

*"I'm sorry, the parents of the young man in that wreck
refuse to donate his liver. They are, however,
giving me an excellent deal on parts for my Porsche."*

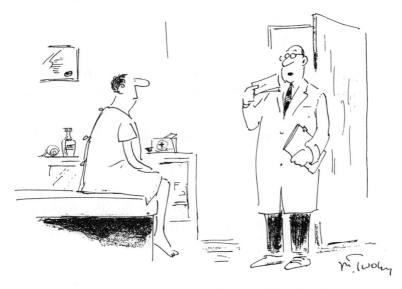

*"Your lab tests are back, John, and I'm just hoping
there was some human error."*

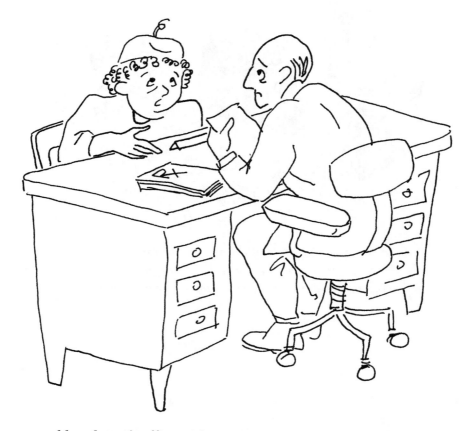

A woman entered her doctor's office with a very grave expression on her face.

"My husband just doesn't seem to have the sexual energy he once had," the woman complained.

"I see," said her physician, with a concerned look on his face. "And just how old is your husband?"

"Seventy-seven."

"Well, in some ways, you just can't blame him, can you? Bodily functions do deteriorate with age. Now tell me, when did you first notice that there was a problem?"

"Last night," she said, "and then again, this morning."

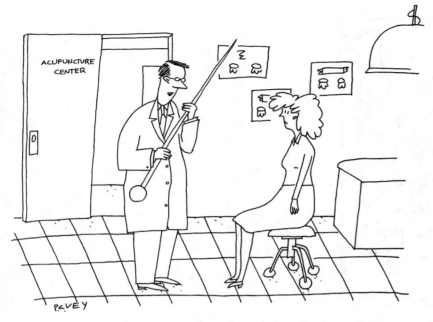

"It's going to hurt more than the two hundred small ones,
but it's much faster."

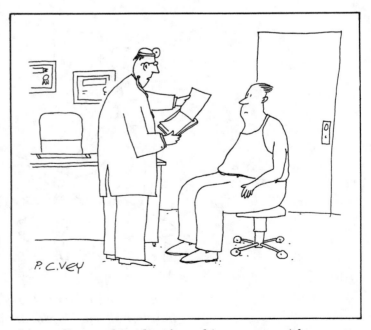

"According to this, there's nothing wrong with you . . .
but then, these are the papers to my house and car."

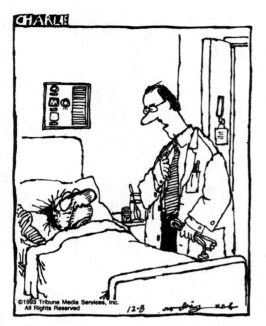

*"You've contracted a virulent strain
of 'Montezuma's revenge, known as
'Montezuma's vindictiveness.'"*

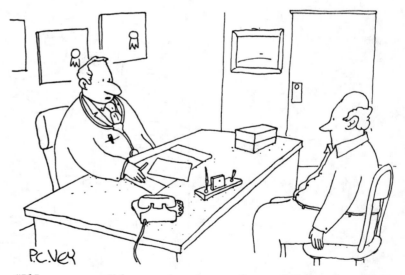

*"If I were you, I'd go to the country for a while . . . but then,
I have a half-million-dollar estate with two swimming pools
and three tennis courts to go to and you don't,
so maybe you'd better stay home."*

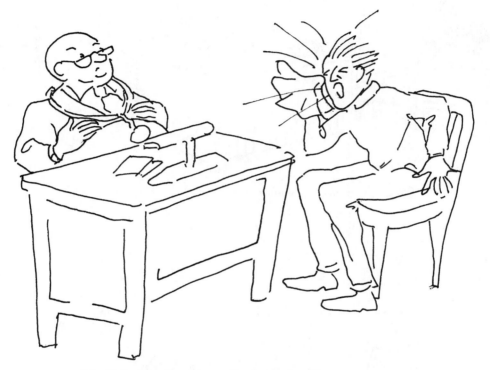

Mr. Baker walked into the doctor's office.
"Is that cough any better today?" the doctor asked.
"Absolutely," said Baker. "I practiced all night."

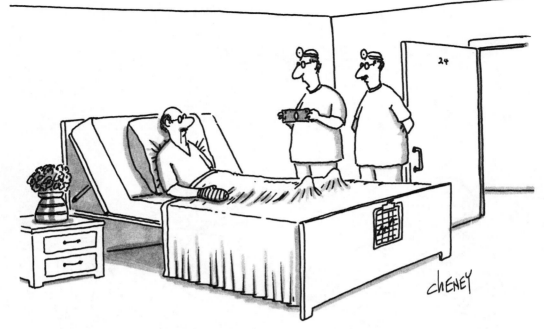

*"**This,** Mr. Brillton, is what we found lodged in your fist."*

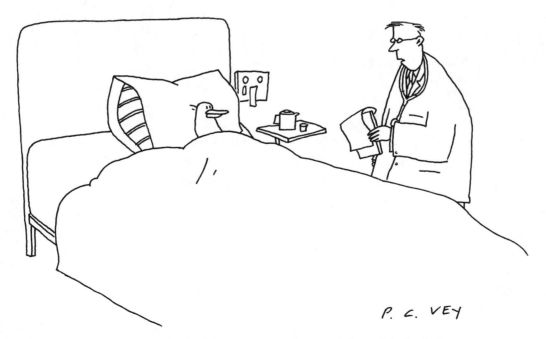

"Let me put it this way— you're a mighty sick duck."

Between a Doc and a Scarred Place

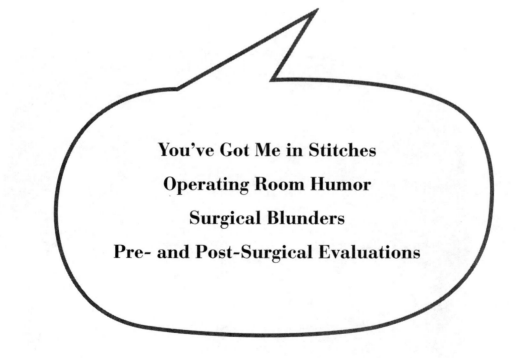

You've Got Me in Stitches

Operating Room Humor

Surgical Blunders

Pre- and Post-Surgical Evaluations

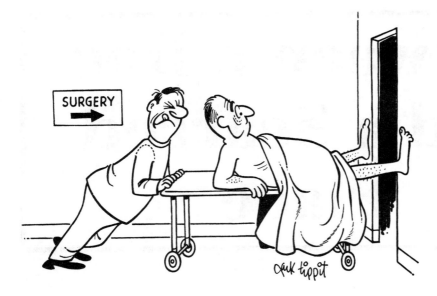

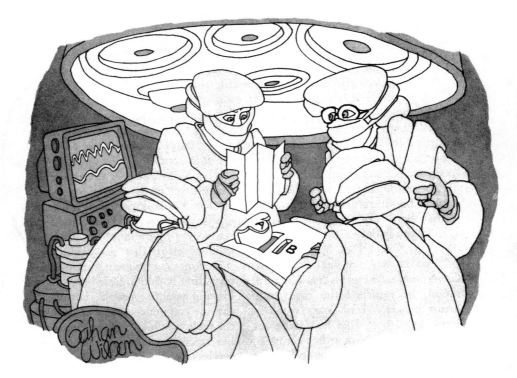

"O.K., now put Tab A into Slot B."

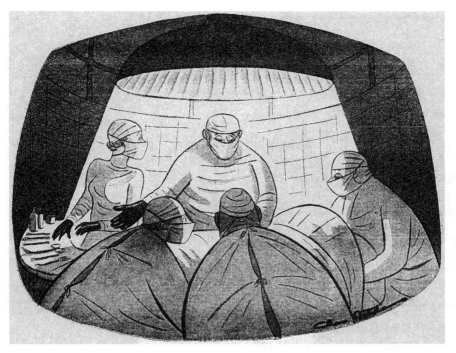

"Scotch Tape."

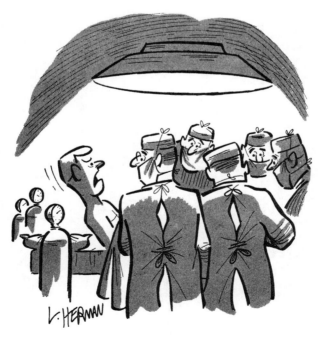

"How do you expect me to sleep with that light on?"

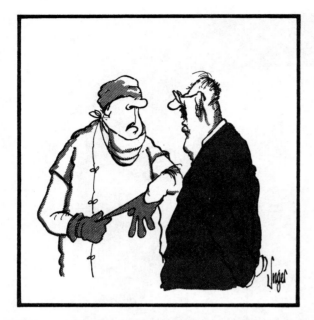

"Your wife is still under the anesthetic and, from what I've heard, this would be a good time to see her."

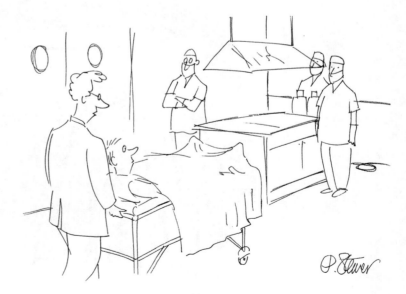

"It only looks like a salad bar."

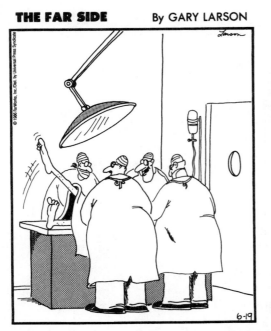

THE FAR SIDE   By GARY LARSON

"Whoa! That was a good one! Try it, Hobbs—
just poke his brain right where my finger is."

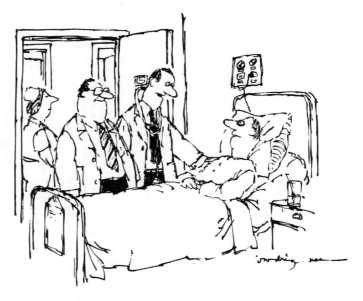

*"I'll do your actual sex-change surgery,
and Dr. Feldstein here, a psychiatrist,
will take care of your desire to be a nymphomaniac."*

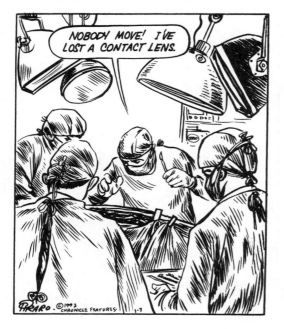

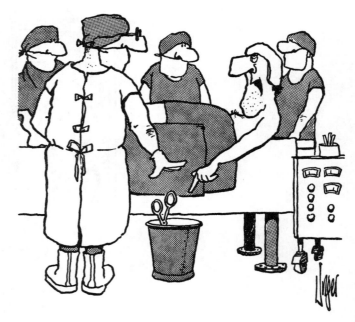

"What was that?"

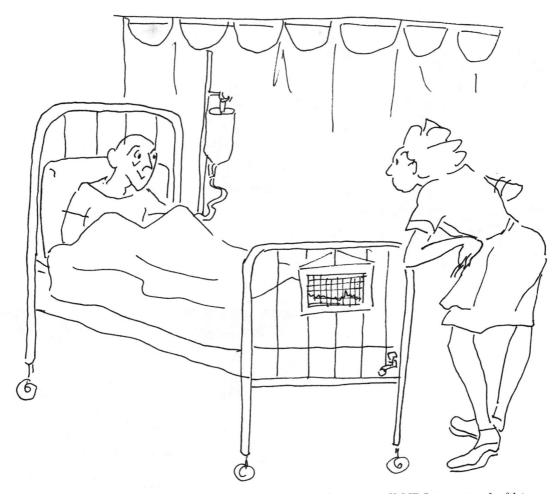

George, a post-surgical patient, who was still NPO, inquired of his nurse, "Do you think I could have an extra intravenous bottle today?"

"Why?" the nurse asked.

"Well, I was thinking of asking someone to lunch."

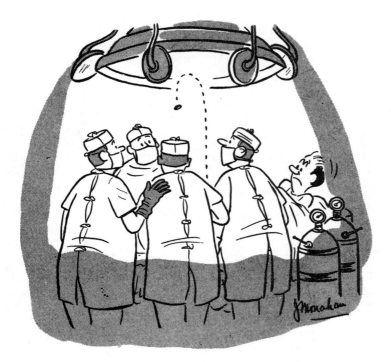

"Heads!"

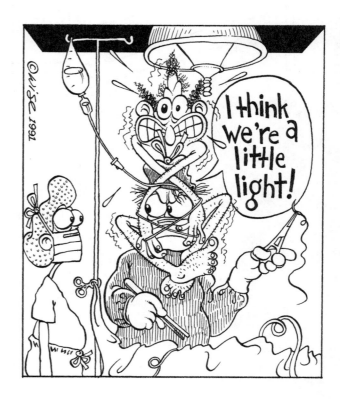

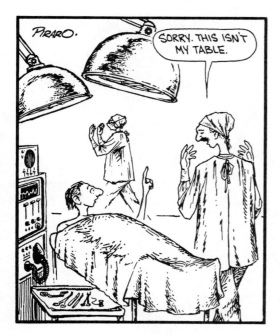

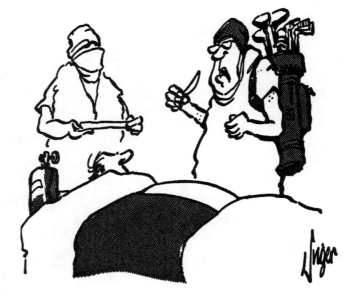

"This shouldn't take too long!"

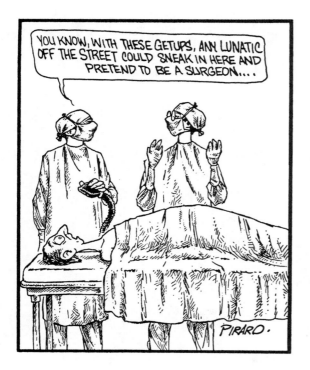

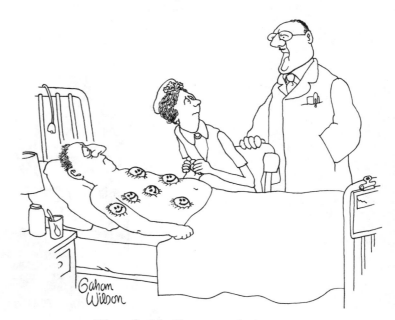

*"I'm afraid all we can do is operate
and hope they don't continue to spread!"*

By GARY LARSON

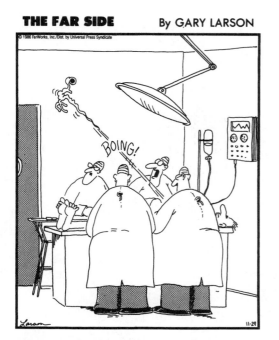

"Whoa! Watch where that thing lands
—we'll probably need it."

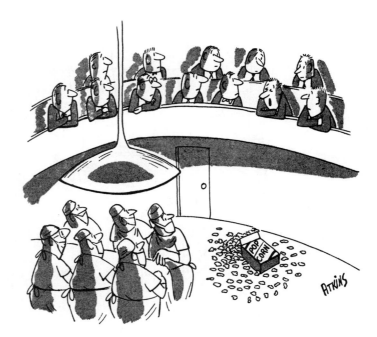

"Sorry!"

27

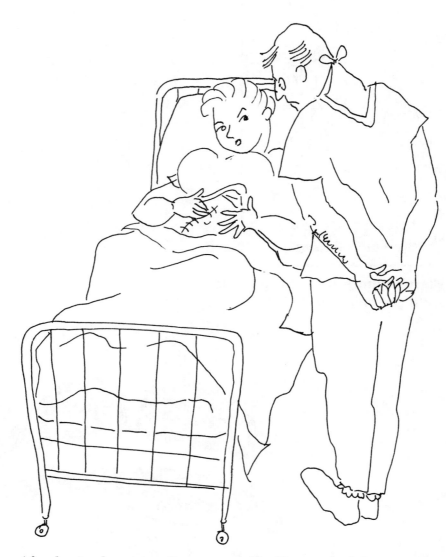

After having her appendix removed, Ms. Pierce asked the surgeon,
"Do you think the scar will show?"
"That," the doctor replied, "is entirely up to you."

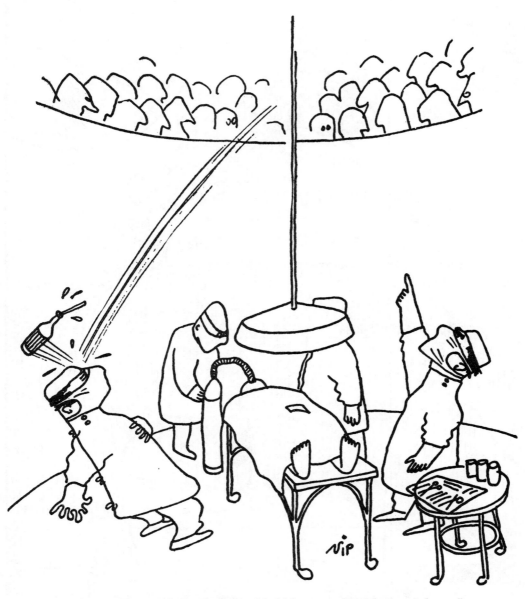

"*If one of you doctors thinks he can do a better job . . .*"

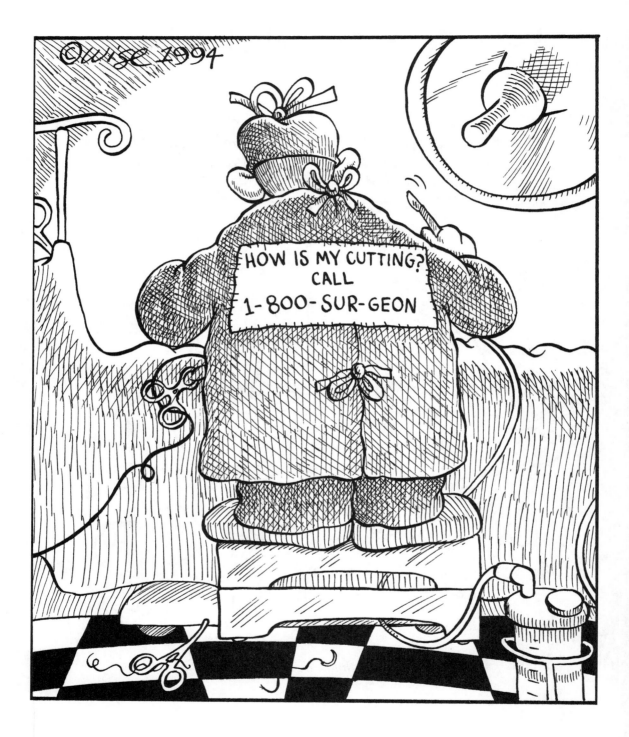

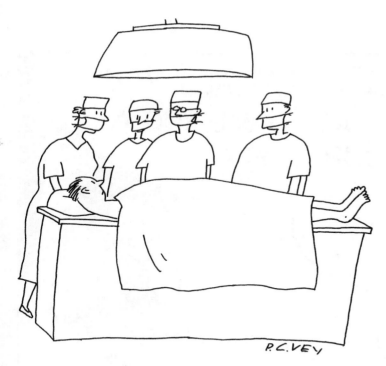

"O.K.—Which one of us is talking now?"

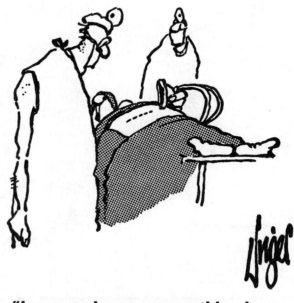

**"Leave a clamp or something in me.
I could really use the money."**

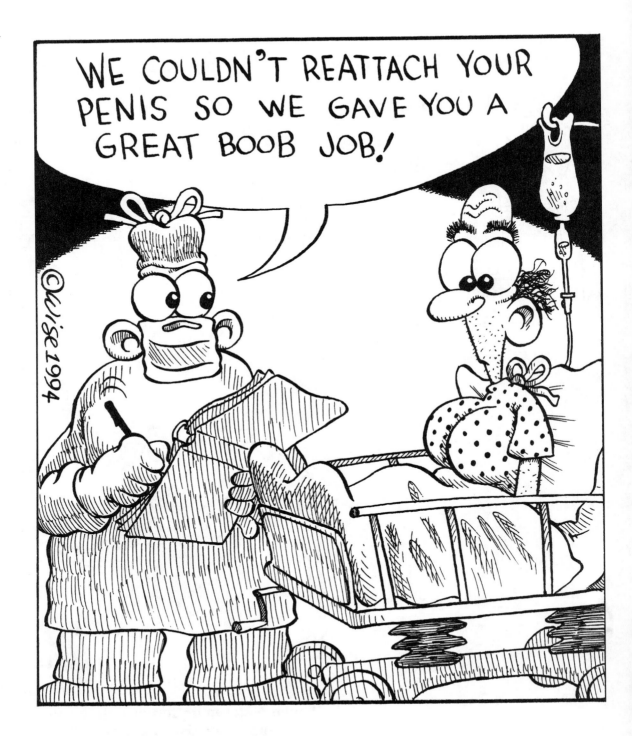

On the Couch

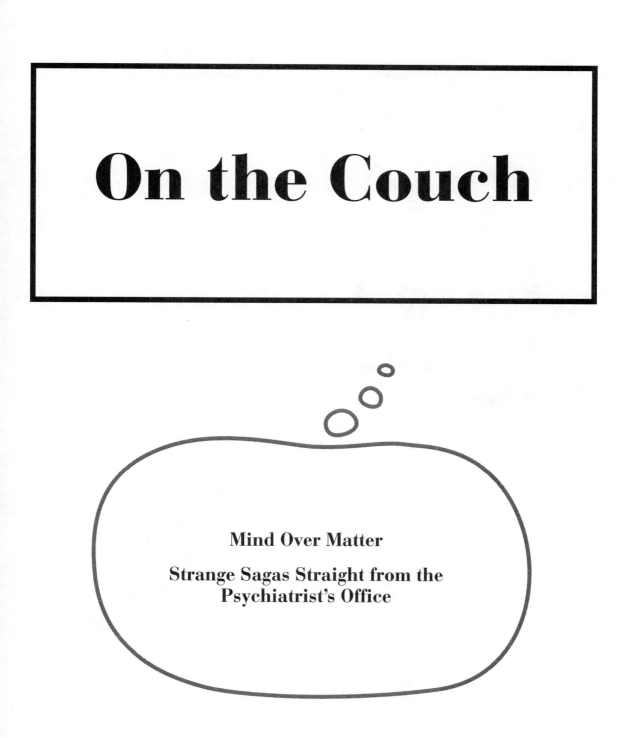

Mind Over Matter

**Strange Sagas Straight from the
Psychiatrist's Office**

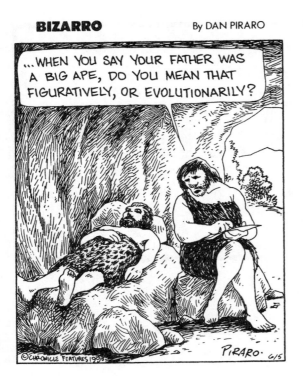

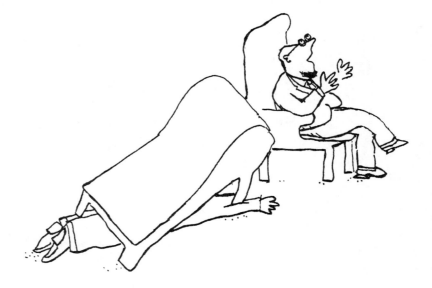

"Basically, Mr. Wilson, what I seem to be hearing you say is 'help'!"

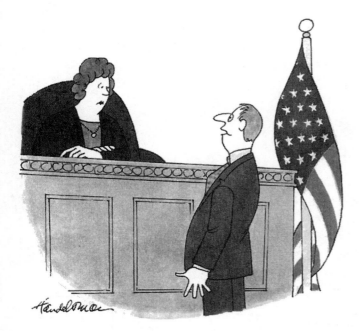

"Now that I've swung back to depression,
I'm truly sorry for what I did when I was manic."

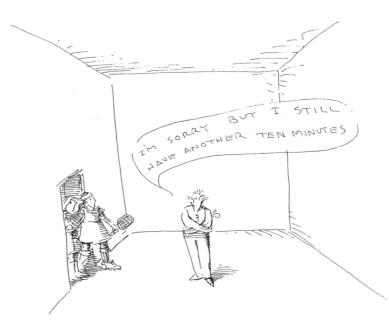

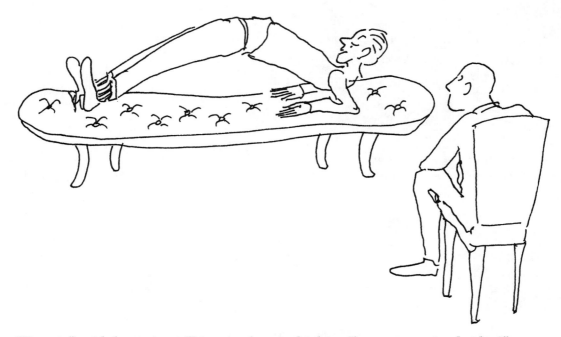

"Doctor," said the patient, "I just can't stop thinking I'm a suspension bridge!"
"Good Lord," said the doctor, "what's come over you?"
"Well, so far—two trucks, five cars, and a Greyhound bus."

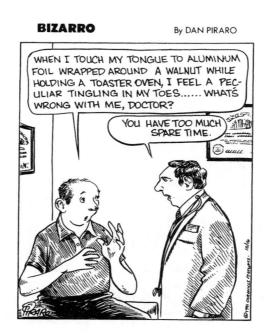

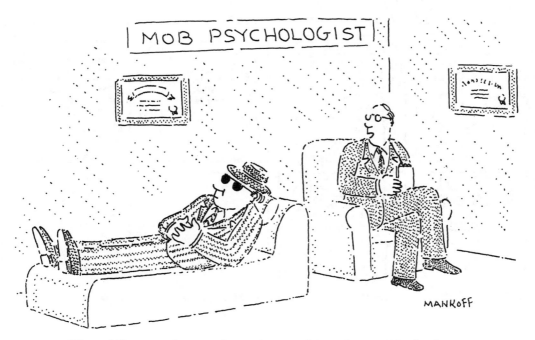

"So, while extortion, racketeering, and murder may be bad acts, they don't make you a bad person."

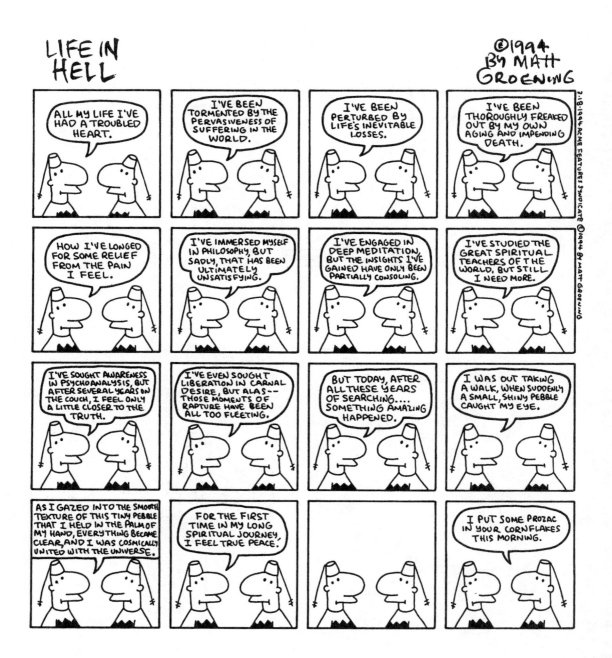

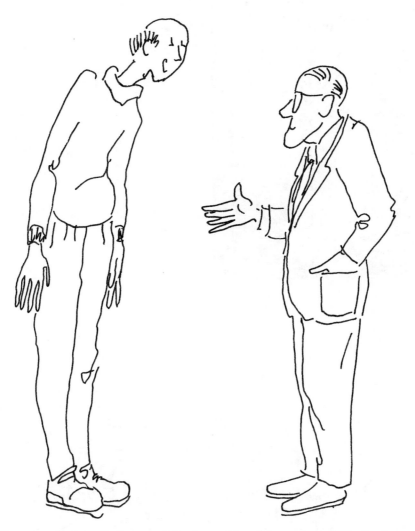

"Congratulations," the psychiatrist said to his patient. "You're cured!"

"Big deal," the patient complained. "Before I came to you for therapy, I thought I was John F. Kennedy. Now, I'm a nobody!"

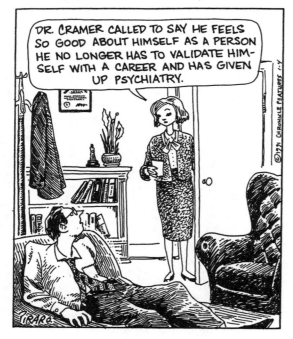

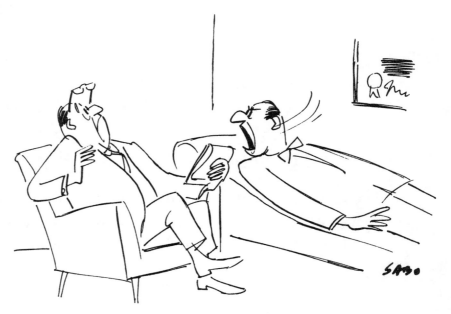

"You keep my dear mother out of this!"

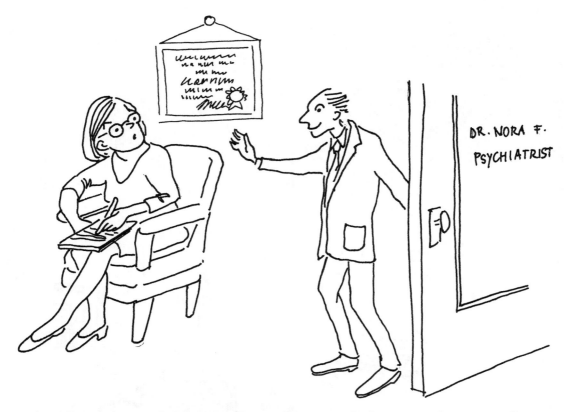

"I feel like a new man," the schizophrenic patient said after years of treatment."
"Anyone I know?" asked his doctor.

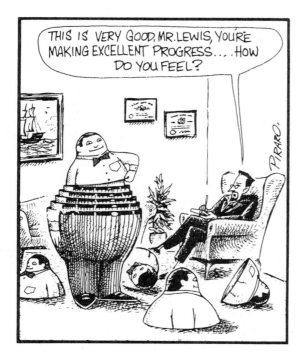

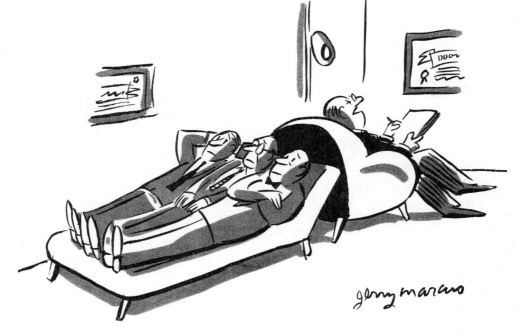

"First, let me explain how group therapy works."

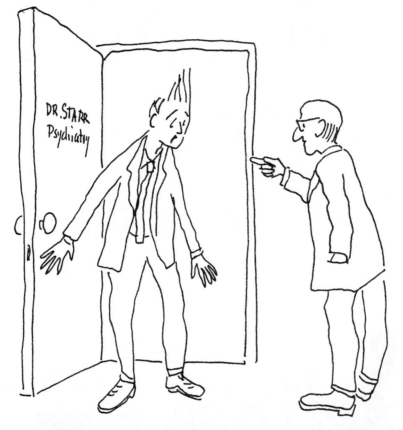

The young man entered the psychiatrist's office and said, "I just don't know how to explain it. I have this bizarre feeling that sometimes I'm a teepee and the rest of the time I'm a wigwam. Do you have any idea what could be wrong with me?"

"You're too tents."

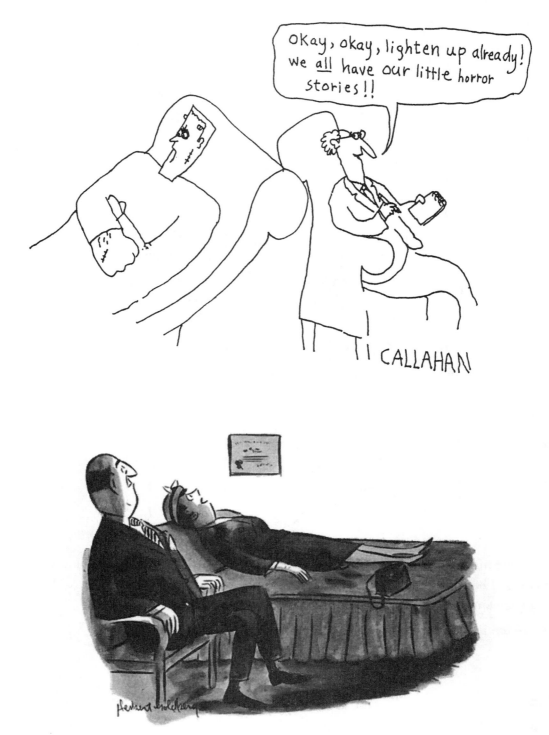

"Your ceiling could stand painting."

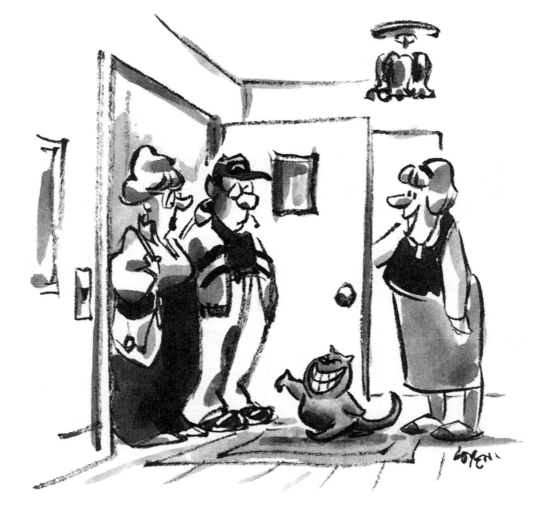

*"Before Prozac, she **loathed** company."*

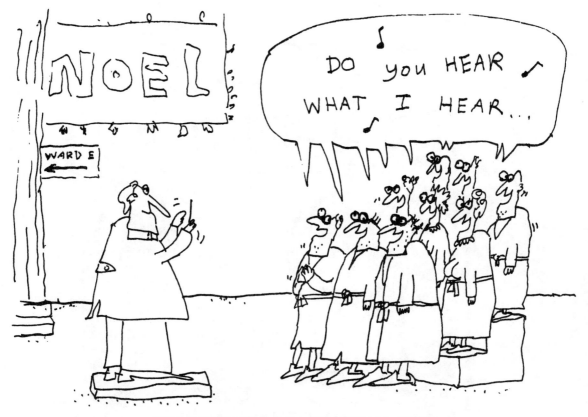

THE SCHIZOPHRENIC CHRISTMAS CHOIR

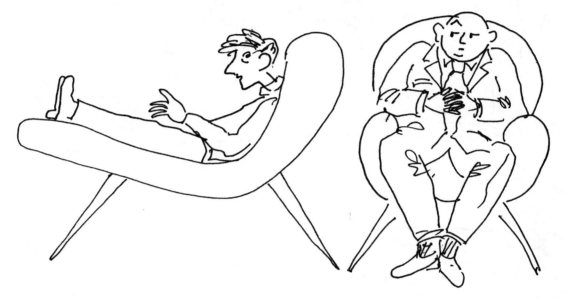

"I think I'm beginning to understand the root of your problem," the psychiatrist said to his patient. "Now tell me, why exactly do you hate your mother?"

"I don't," said the patient. "In fact, I love my mother very, very much."

"Look," the doctor said adamantly, "If you're not going to cooperate with me, I'll never be able to help you."

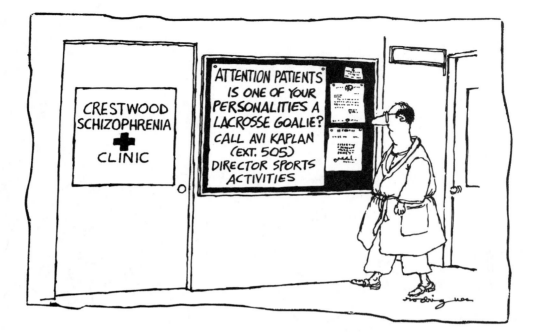

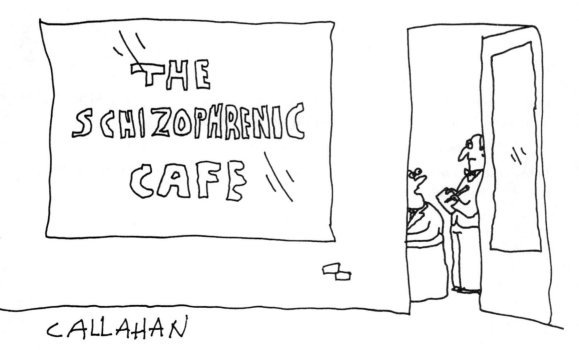

CALLAHAN

"I'll have what I'm having."

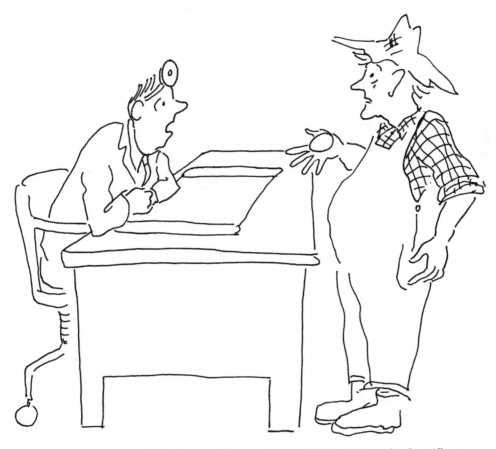

Patient: "Doctor, my little brother is really crazy. He thinks he's a chicken!"

Doctor: "How long has this been going on?"

Patient: "For about five years."

Doctor: "Oh my gosh! Why have you waited so long to come for medical attention?"

Patient: "We needed the eggs!"

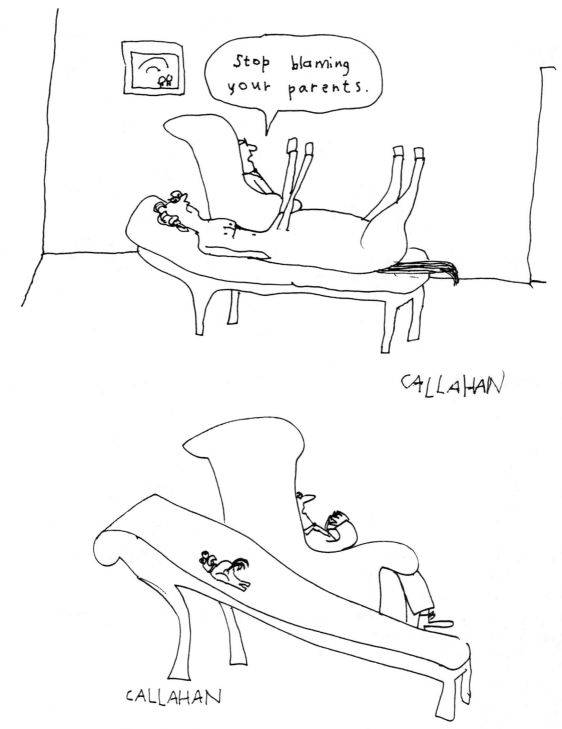

*"Do you **want** a cracker, or do you **need** a cracker?"*

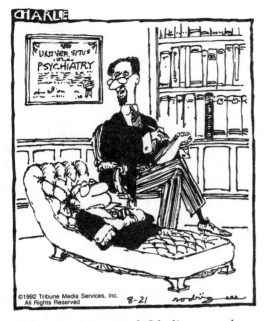

*"If you're interested, I believe you have
sufficient phobias, manias, and delusions to
qualify for a handicap parking plate."*

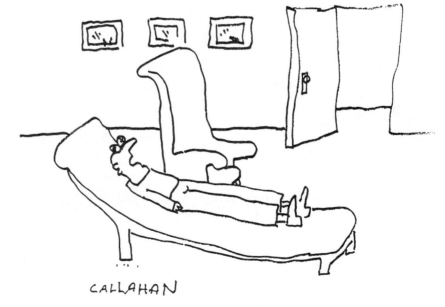

CALLAHAN

"I'd like to talk about my abandonment issues."

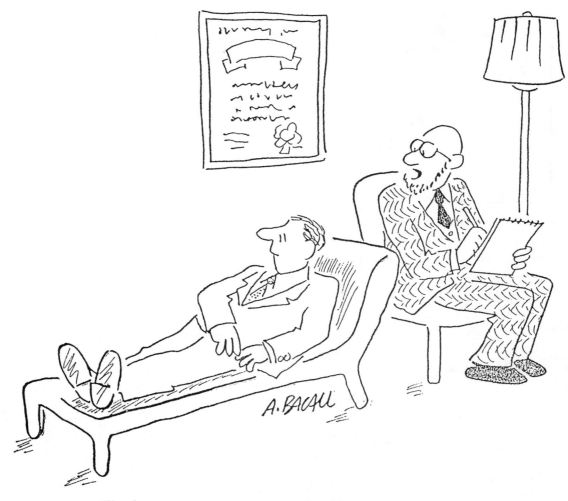

"You have to get out more. Meet people. Make new enemies."

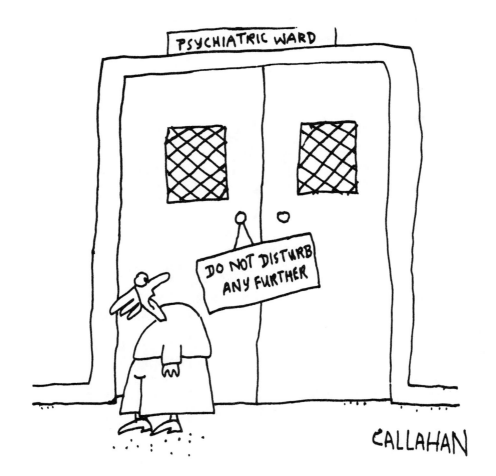

Within Humorous Limits

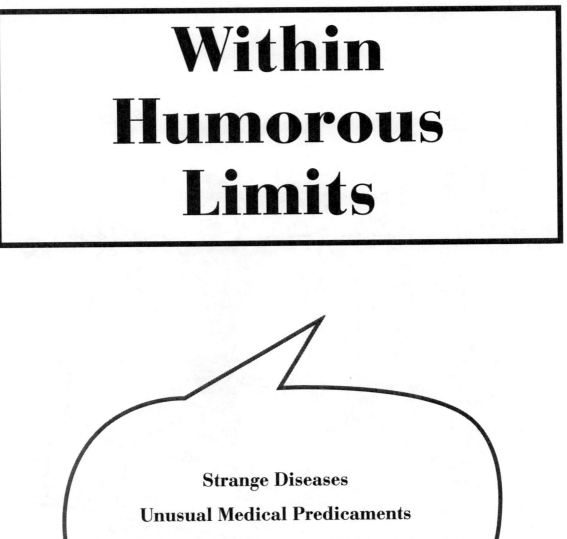

Strange Diseases

Unusual Medical Predicaments

Bizarre Medical and Hospital Encounters

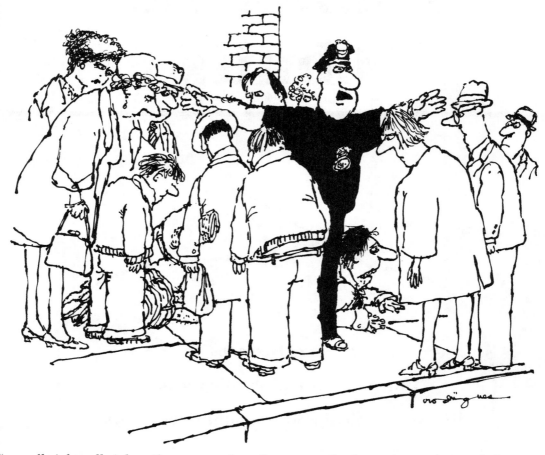

"... all right, all right—I'm sure you've all seen somebody getting an enema before ..."

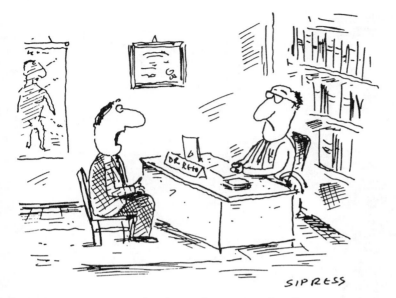

SIPRESS

I want to have that operation I
*heard about on **All Things Considered**.*

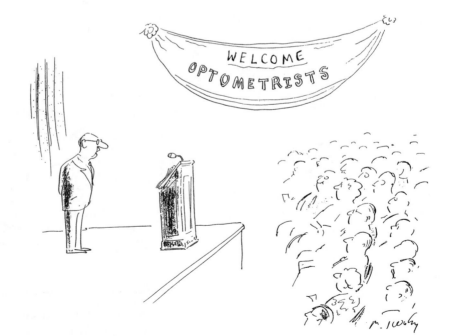

WELCOME OPTOMETRISTS

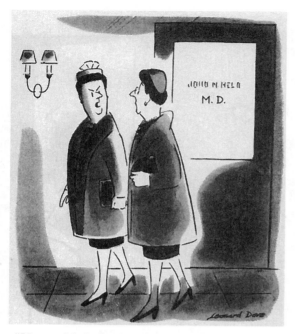

"He couldn't find a thing wrong with me—
the quack."

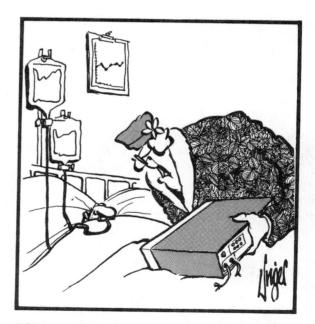

**"Show me what to press if I want to
record a movie after I've gone to bed."**

THE FAR SIDE   By GARY LARSON

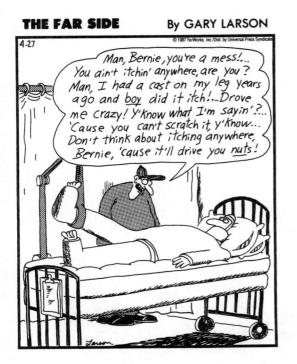

CLOSE TO HOME   JOHN McPHERSON

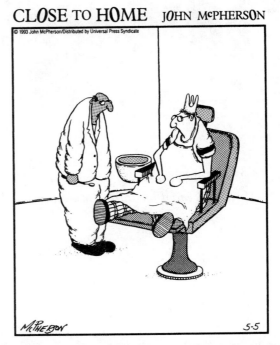

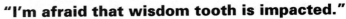

"I'm afraid that wisdom tooth is impacted."

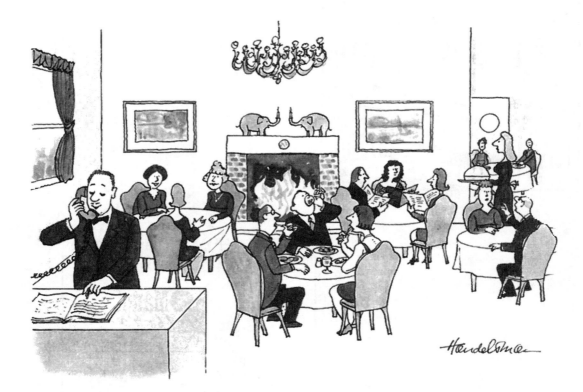

"Certainly. A party of four at seven-thirty in the name of Dr. Jennings. May I ask whether that is an actual medical degree or merely a Ph.D.?"

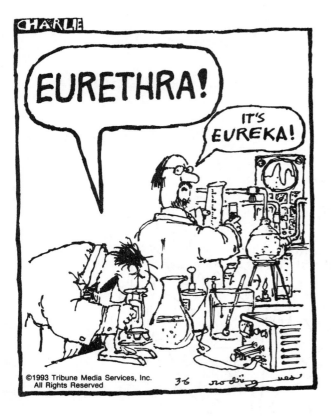

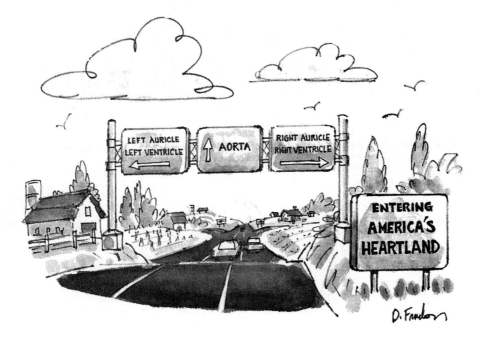

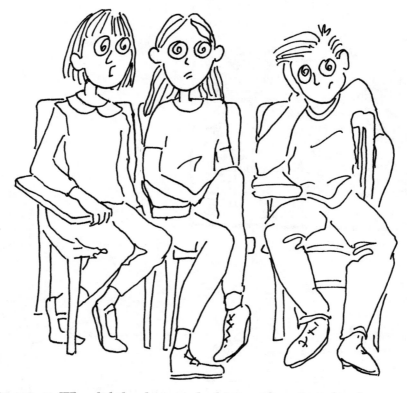

Question: Why did the doctor take his eye chart into the classroom?
Answer: He wanted to check the pupils.

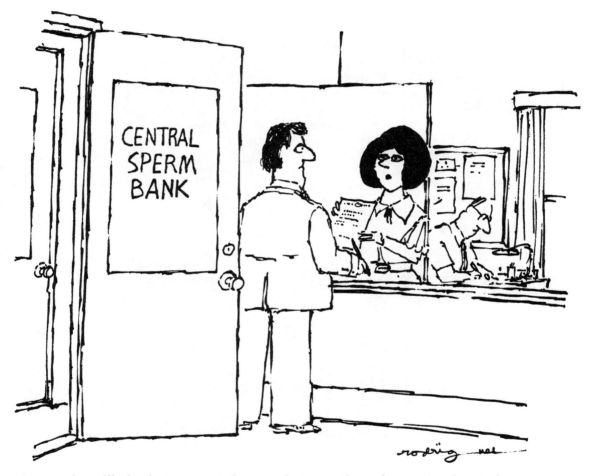

"*. . . and you'll also have to sign this one that says that after you've donated your sperm, you'll still respect us.*"

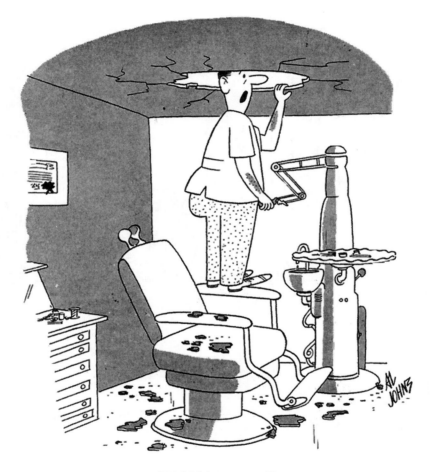

"*Did I hit a nerve?*"

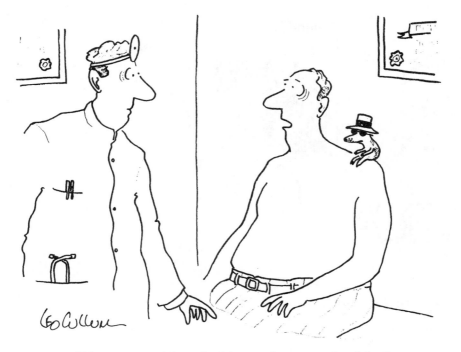

"I have a suspicious looking mole on my shoulder."

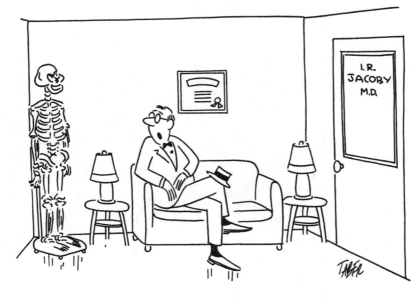

"How long have you been waiting?"

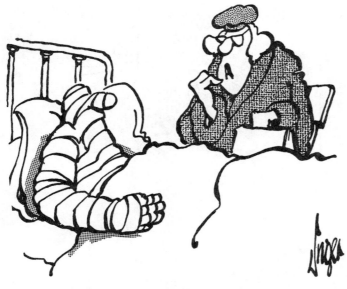

"Oh no! I've broken my nail."

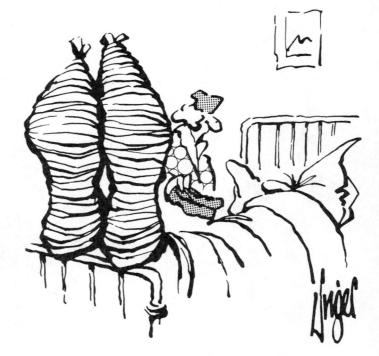

"I brought your slippers."

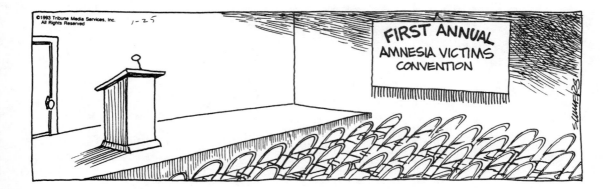

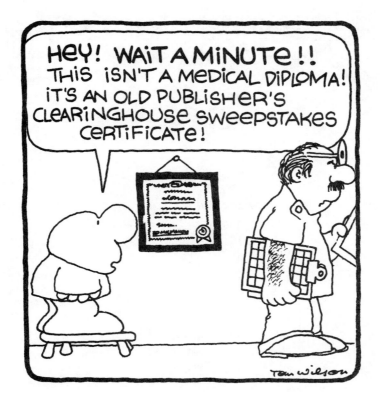

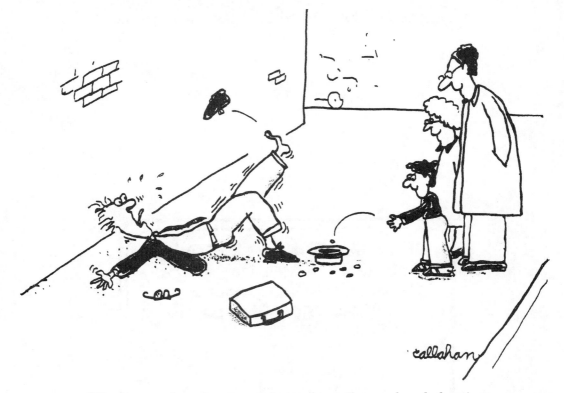

*"Please stop throwing money in my hat—I'm not break dancing,
I'm having a seizure, for heaven's sake!"*

A Bitter Pill to Swallow

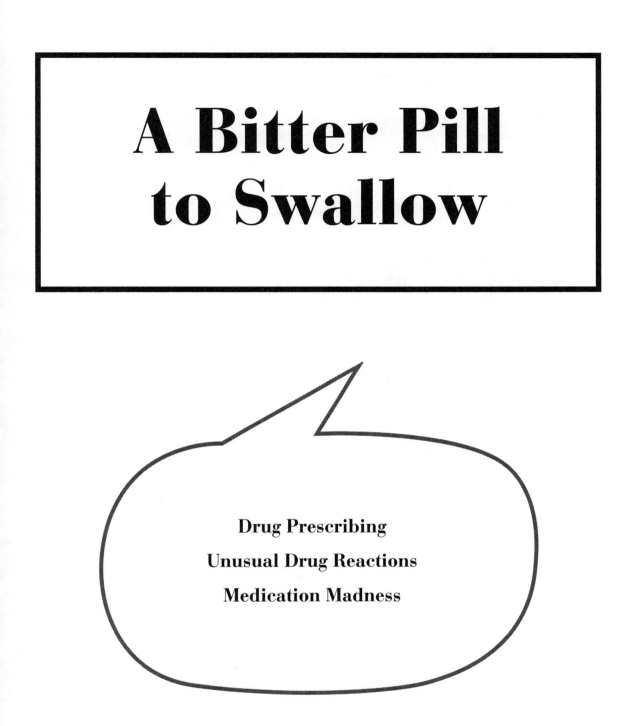

Drug Prescribing

Unusual Drug Reactions

Medication Madness

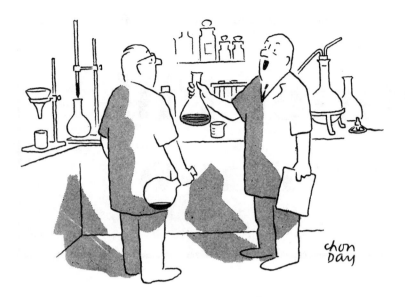

*"It doesn't cure anything, but the side effects
are out of this world."*

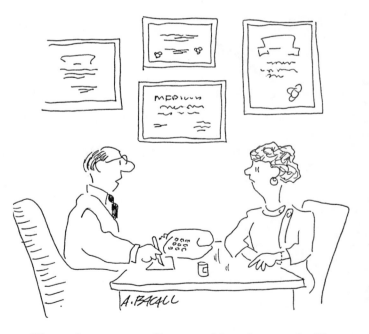

*"I'm going to prescribe something that works like
aspirin but costs much, much more."*

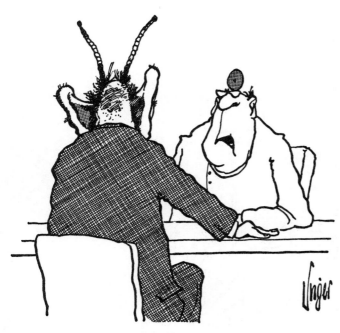

**"If you remember,
I did mention possible side-effects."**

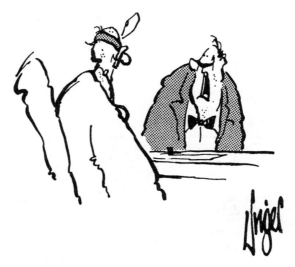

**"And don't give me any of those local anesthetics.
Get me the imported stuff."**

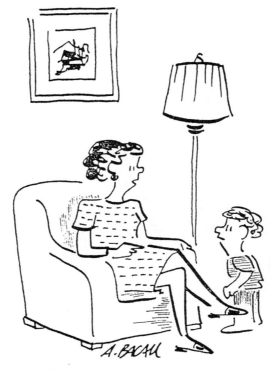

"Yes, when I was your age, all my friends used drugs,
but they were all acne medications."

FRANK & ERNEST® by Bob Thaves

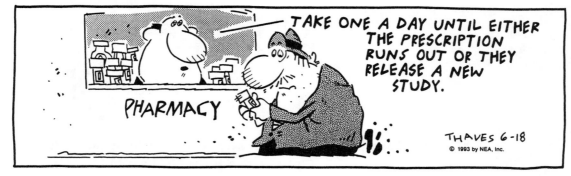

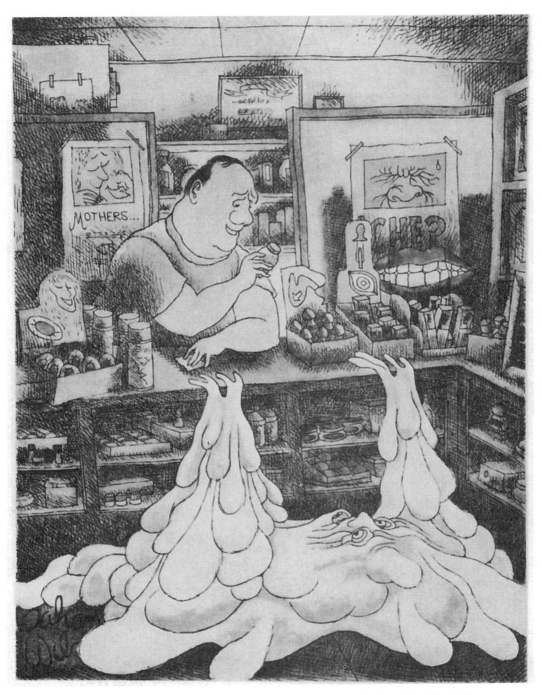

*"My goodness, Mr. Merryweather, we certainly **did** make a boo-boo with that prescription of yours!"*

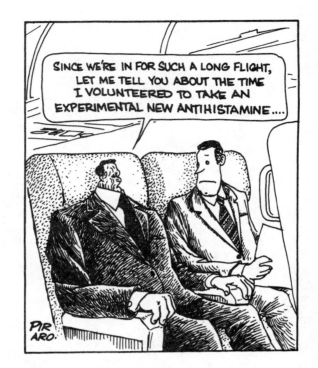

ERNEST / BOB THAVES

PHARMACY

THIS IS TIME-RELEASED
MEDICINE. IT DOESN'T
GO OFF UNTIL
YOUR CHECK CLEARS.

-- THAVES 1·3·87

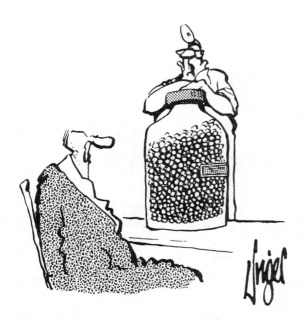

**"I hope you're not one of those people
who have trouble swallowing pills."**

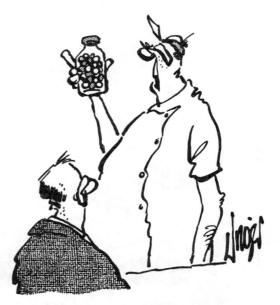

**"I'm not sure what these are,
but take them for a couple of weeks
and let me know how you feel."**

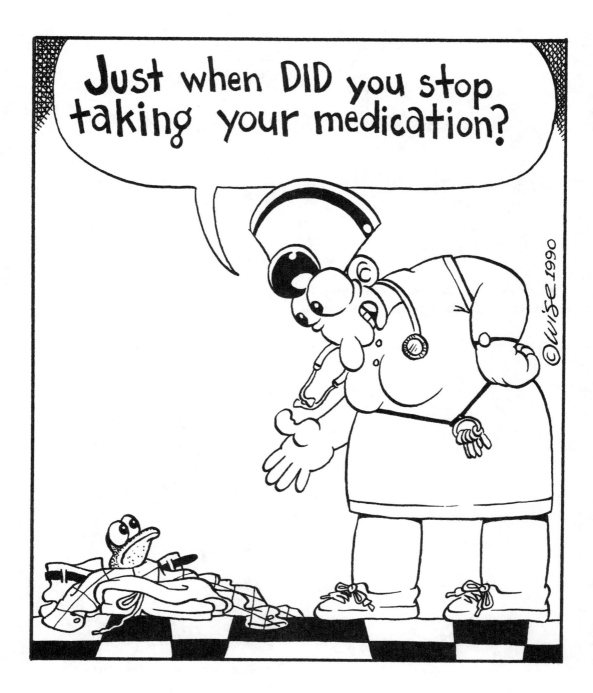

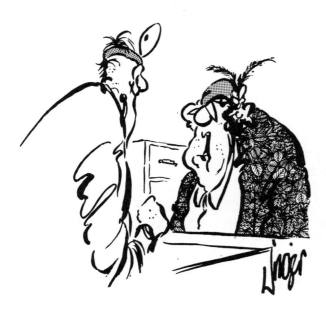

"I feel a lot better since I ran out of those pills you gave me."

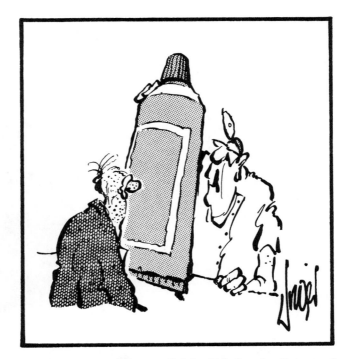

"Rub this on everything within 50 feet of your house."

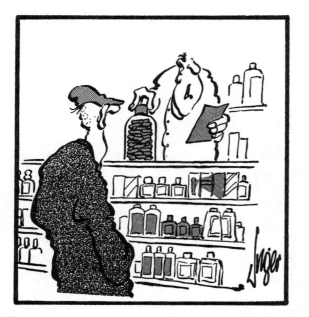

"Take one capsule tonight, and if there's no improvement by tomorrow morning, take the whole bottle."

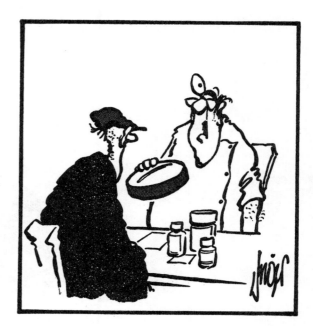

"I want you to take one of these with water every four years."

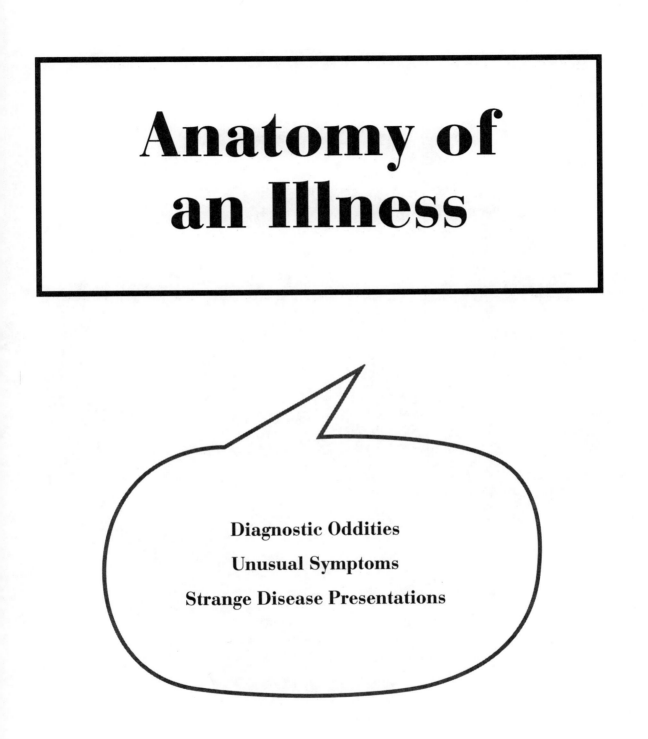

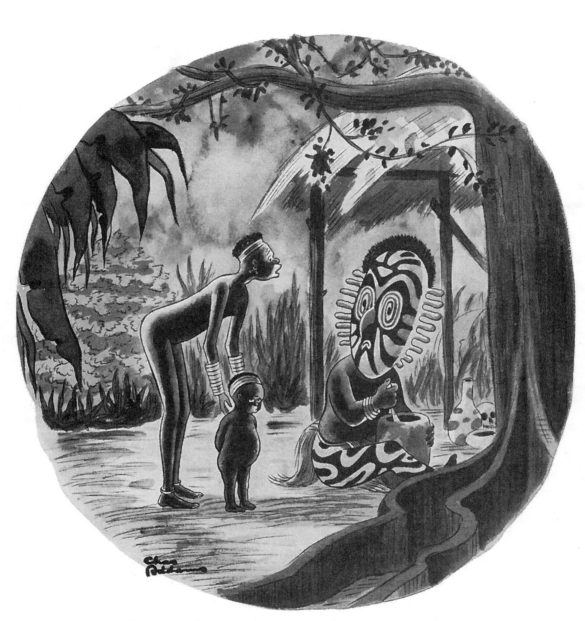

"I'm worried about him, Doctor. He won't eat anybody."

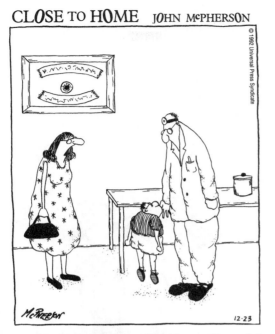

© 1992 Universal Press Syndicate

12-23

"I'm concerned about his thumbsucking."

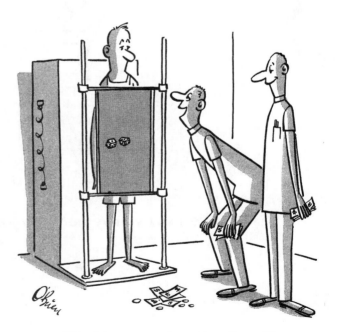

"Would you cough again, please?"

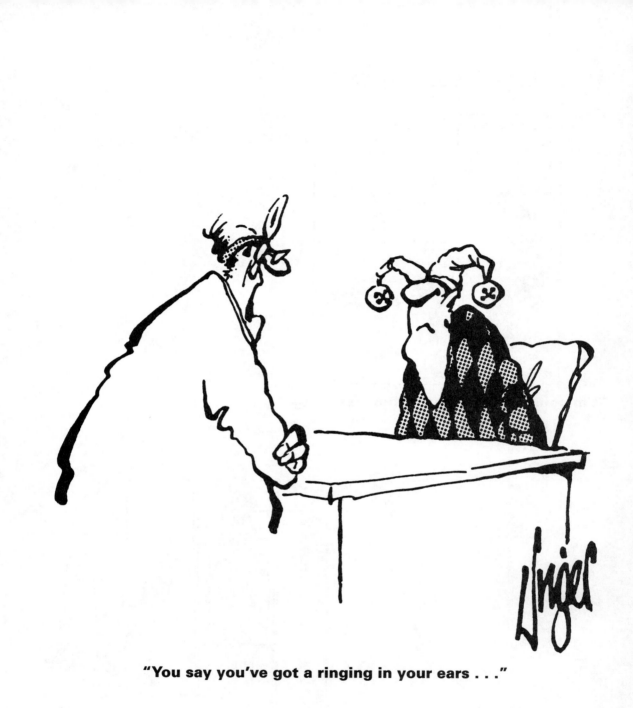

"You say you've got a ringing in your ears . . ."

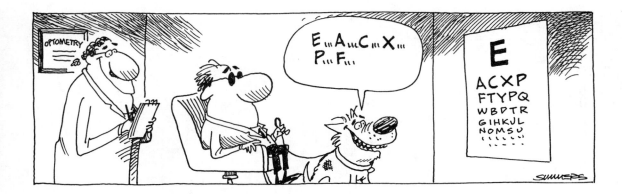

FRANK & ERNEST® by Bob Thaves

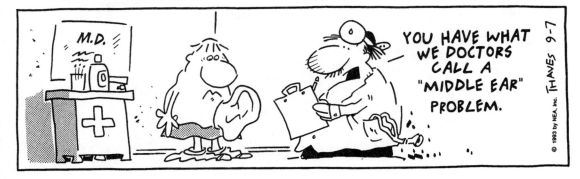

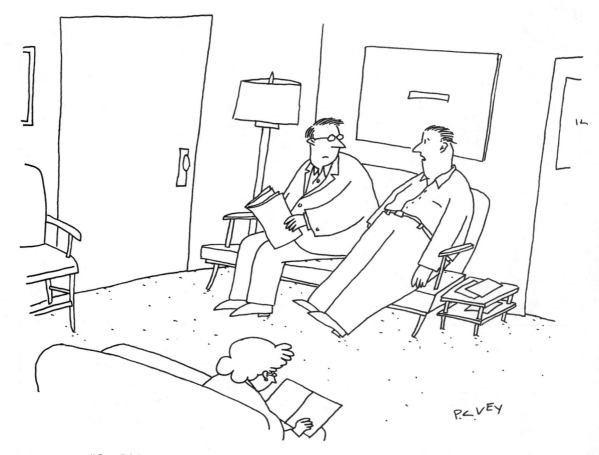

"*Could I see the doctor before you? I think rigor mortis is setting in.*"

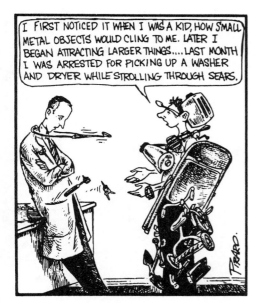

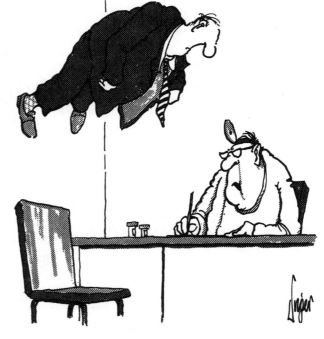

"I'll give you something for gas!"

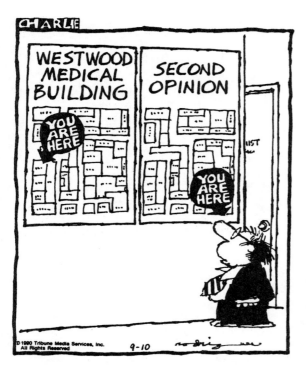

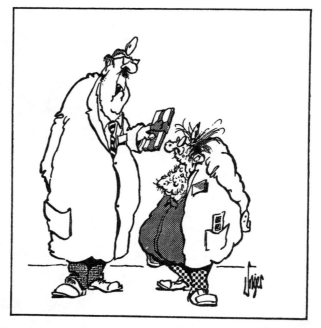

"And in recognition of your 20 years of loyal service in the x-ray department . . ."

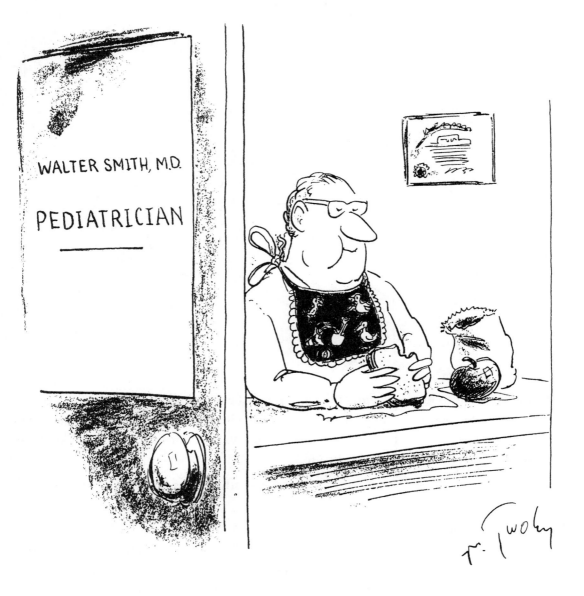

WALTER SMITH, M.D.

PEDIATRICIAN

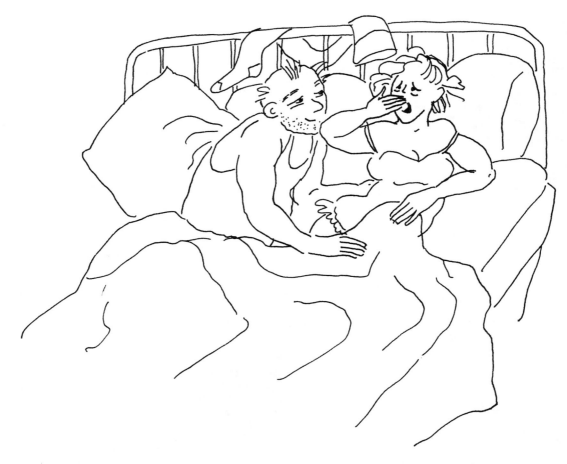

Mr. Childers went to his physician and learned that he only had ten hours left to live. Upon hearing the bad news, he rushed home to his wife and said, "Honey, let's go to bed and make passionate love. I don't have much longer to live, but I'm going to make these the ten most memorable hours of your life."

Once they were undressed, his beloved wife did everything that he had ever wanted a woman to do.

When they were finished, Mr. Childers asked her to do it once again. His wife knew it would take a great deal of stamina, but she obliged. When they were finished, it was three o'clock in the morning and the woman was spent. As she lay flat on her back, her husband asked her for still one more session of passionate lovemaking.

Looking him squarely in the eye, his wife said, "Sure—what do you care? You don't have to get up in the morning!"

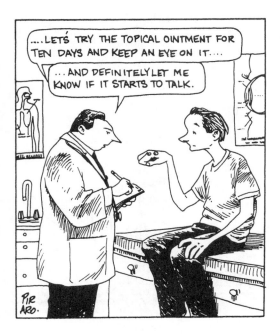

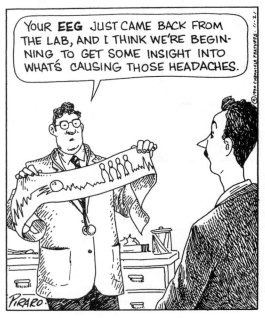

89

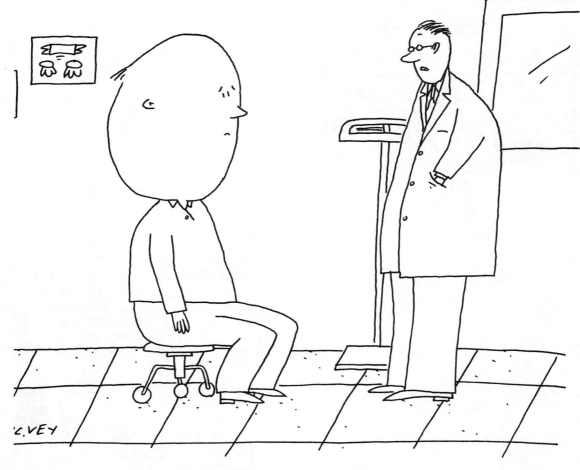

"*Where does it hurt?*"

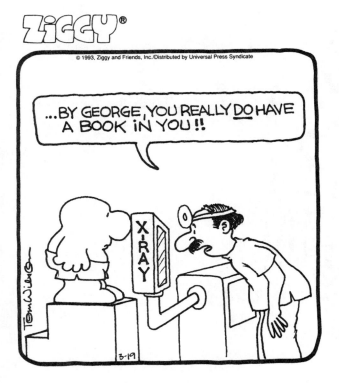

ZiGGY®

...BY GEORGE, YOU REALLY DO HAVE A BOOK IN YOU!!

X-RAY

3-19

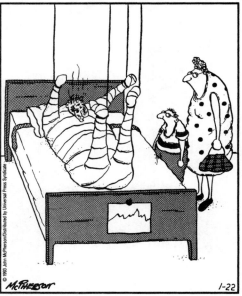

CLOSE TO HOME   JOHN McPHERSON

"Are you gonna make me return the chemistry set?"

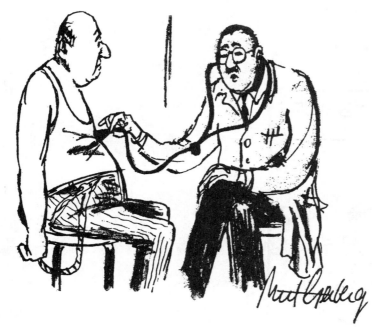

"Okay, now start it up again."

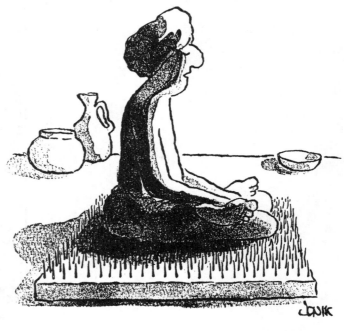

"...OUCH...OUCH...OUCH...OUCH..."

Under My Skin

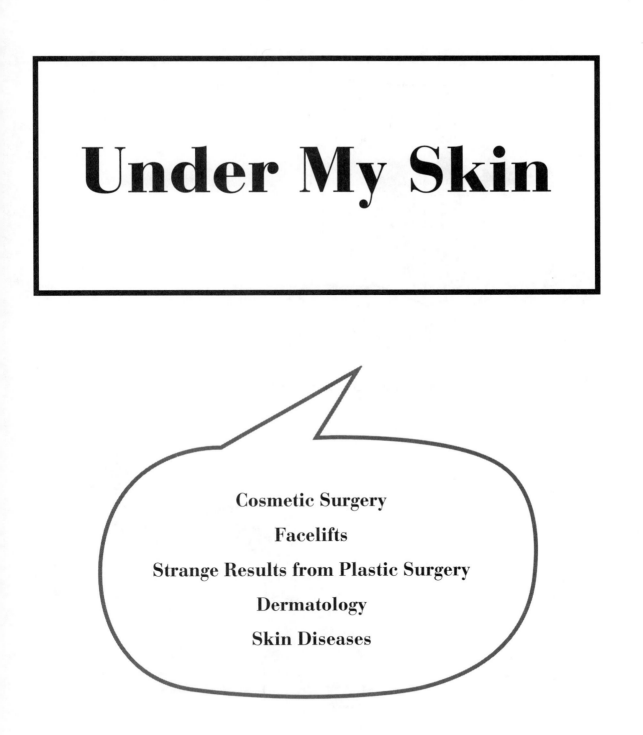

Cosmetic Surgery

Facelifts

Strange Results from Plastic Surgery

Dermatology

Skin Diseases

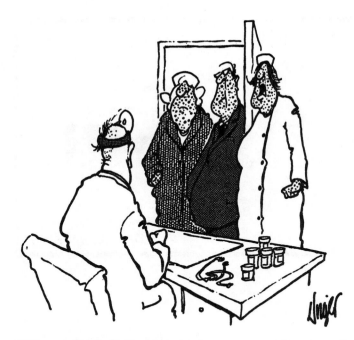

"Mr. and Mrs. Roberts to see you, Doctor."

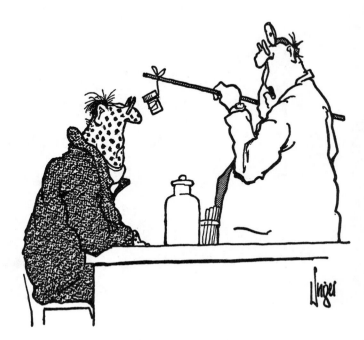

"Here, don't touch the stick."

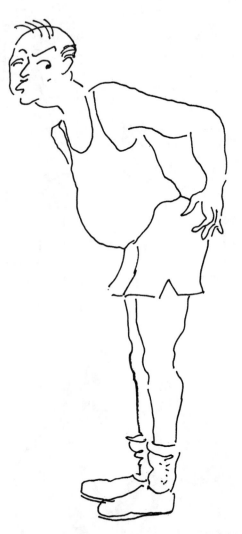

Question: What's the difference between an itch and an allergy?
Answer: A $50 office visit.

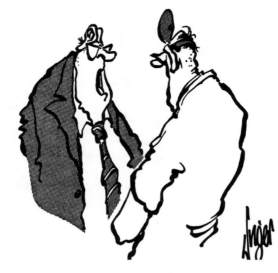

"I like the facelift, but my wife thinks my
ears are a touch too high."

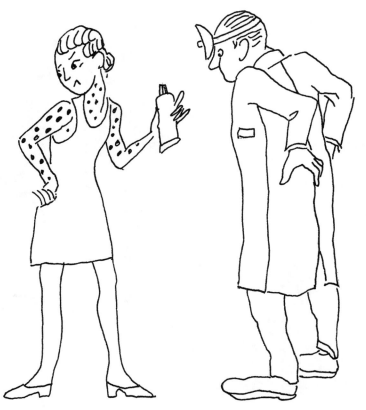

Patient: "Doctor?"

Doctor: "Yes, what is it?"

Patient: "Will this cream you gave me clear up those red spots on my body?"

Doctor: "I never make rash promises!"

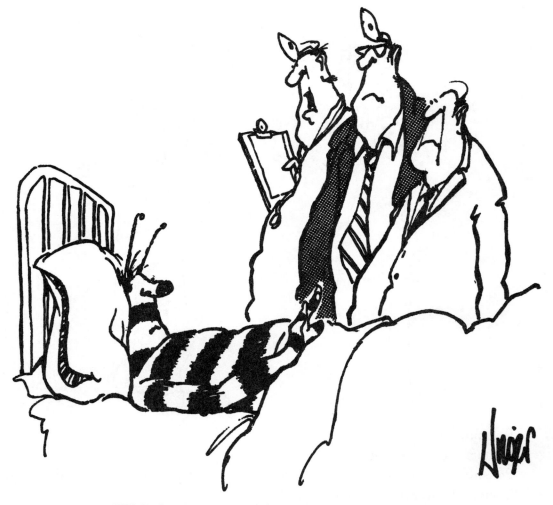

"This is the guy who was stung by a bee."

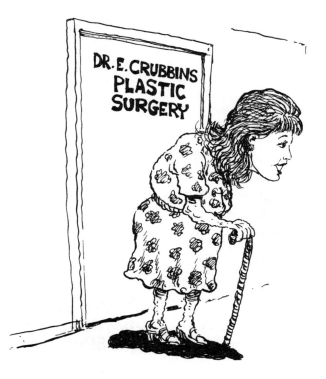

HIPPOSUCTION

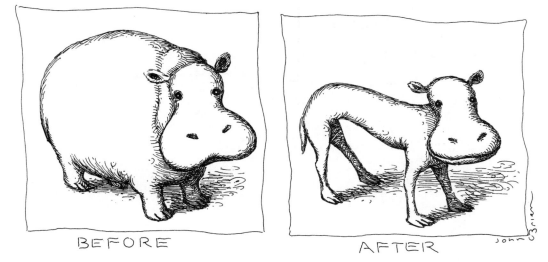

BEFORE

AFTER

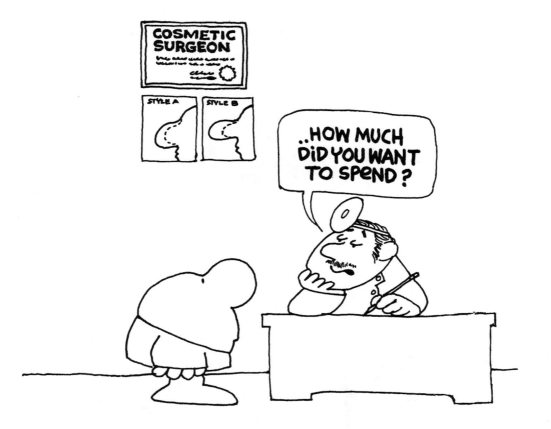

From Here to Maternity

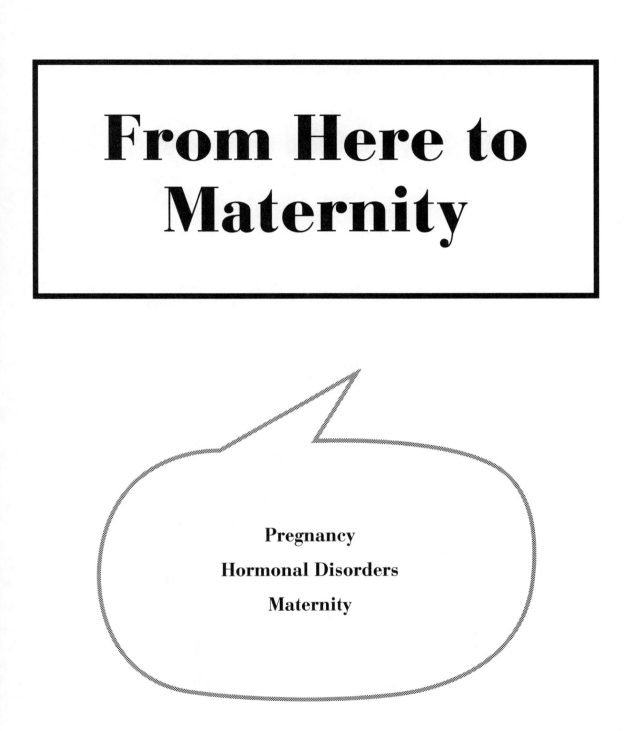

Pregnancy

Hormonal Disorders

Maternity

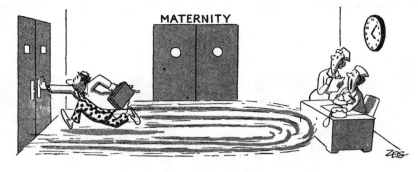

"Forgot his wife."

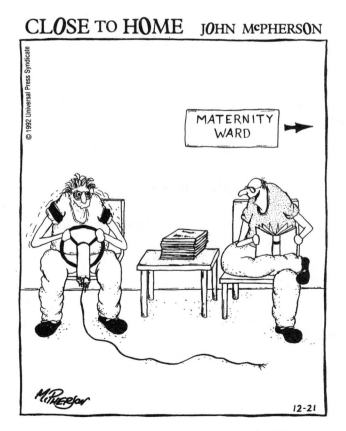

"So, is this your first baby?"

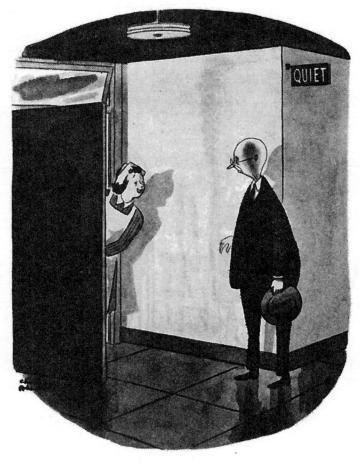

"Congratulations! It's a baby."

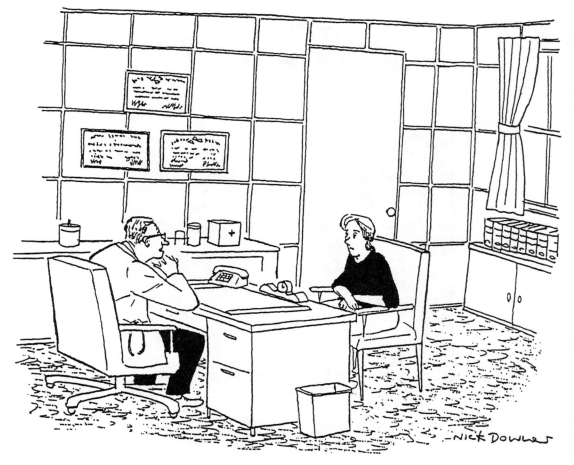

"You're not infertile, Mrs. Simmons.
Perhaps you don't breed well in captivity."

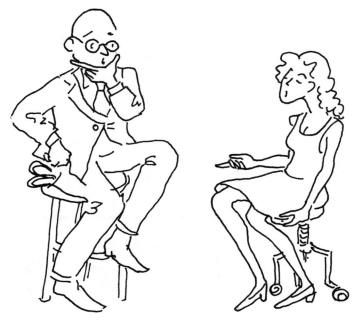

"I am very, very concerned," Lori said to the doctor. "Ever since you told me to use a diaphragm, I've been urinating purple."

"That's very unusual," said the doctor. "What kind of jelly are you using?"

"Grape."

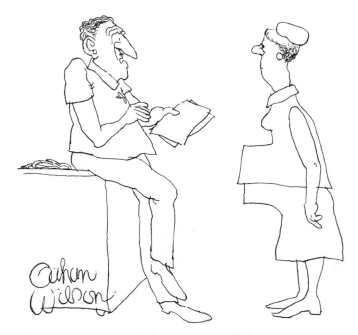

"Of course you realize this may be a difficult birth."

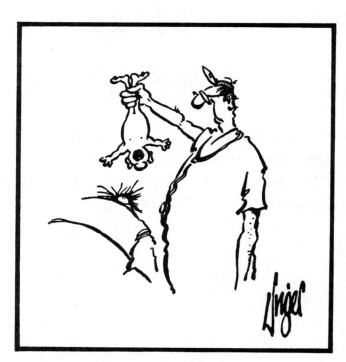

"Get me a lawyer."

CLOSE TO HOME

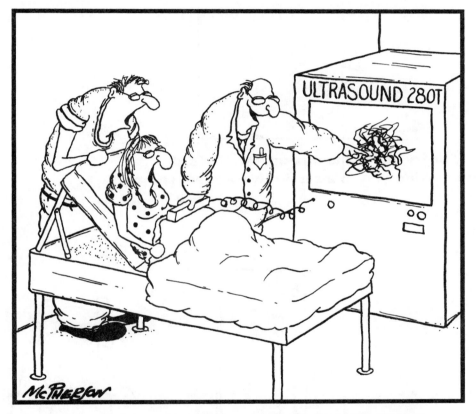

"And here you can clearly see the baby's head and . . .
oh, look! He's wiggling his toes there!"

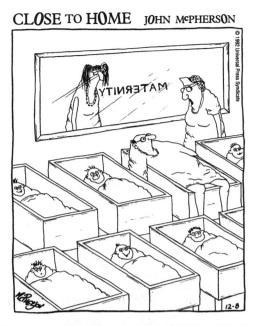

CLOSE TO HOME   JOHN McPHERSON

**"Sorry about the mix-up, Mr. Bixford.
We'll be moving you to a semi-private room shortly."**

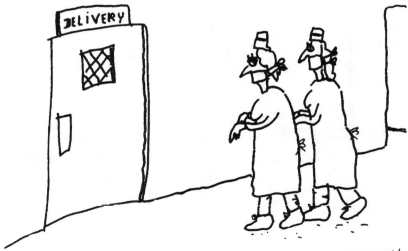

*"Now remember—spank the bottom, cut the cord,
and check the child for weapons."*

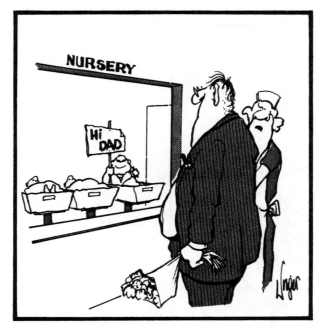

"Congratulations! He seems very bright."

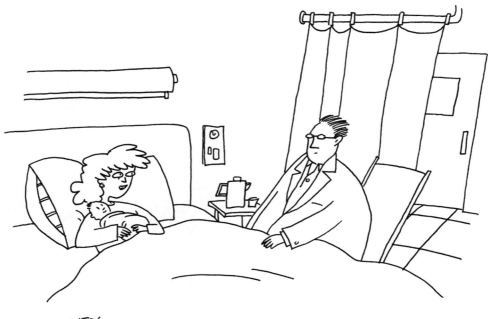

"He's small, I like that in a baby."

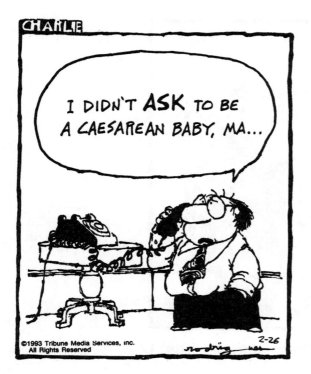

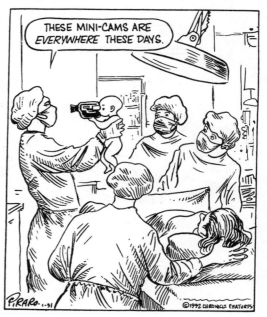

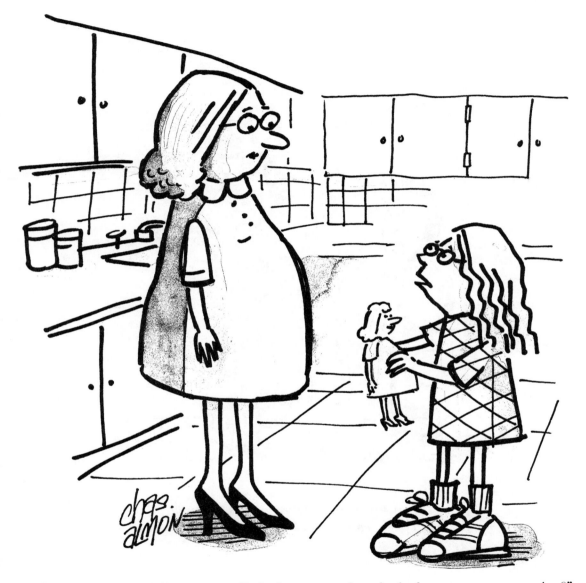

"If these pregnant dolls are so realistic, how come **they** don't throw up every morning?"

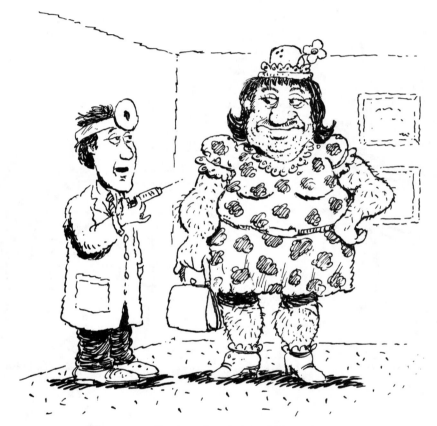

"In my professional opinion, Mrs. Johnson,
we should begin cutting back on your hormone dosage."

Lifestyles of the Sick and Nameless

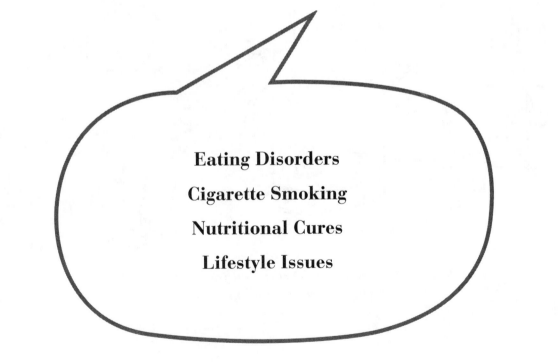

Eating Disorders

Cigarette Smoking

Nutritional Cures

Lifestyle Issues

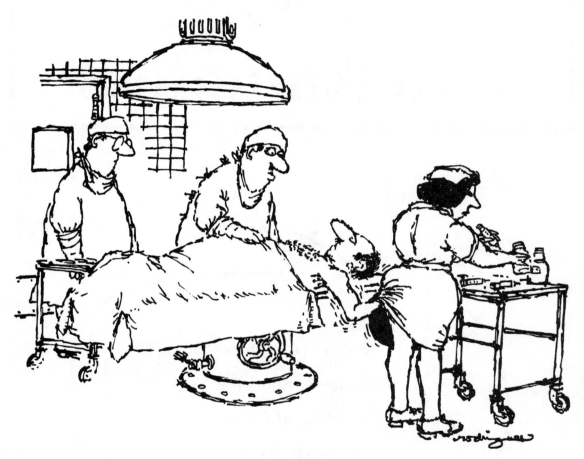

"Mr. Guzman, are you quite sure that you want to go through with this sex-change operation?"

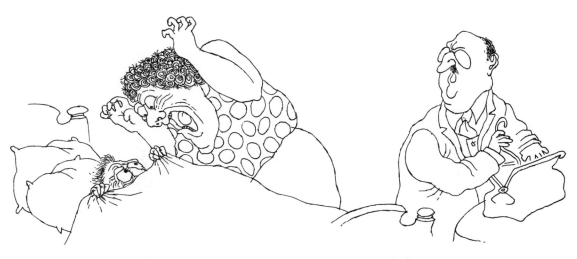

*"Oh, yes, and that's another thing, Mrs. Salzman.
Don't do that anymore to Mr. Salzman."*

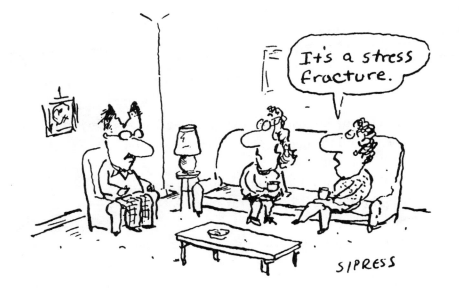

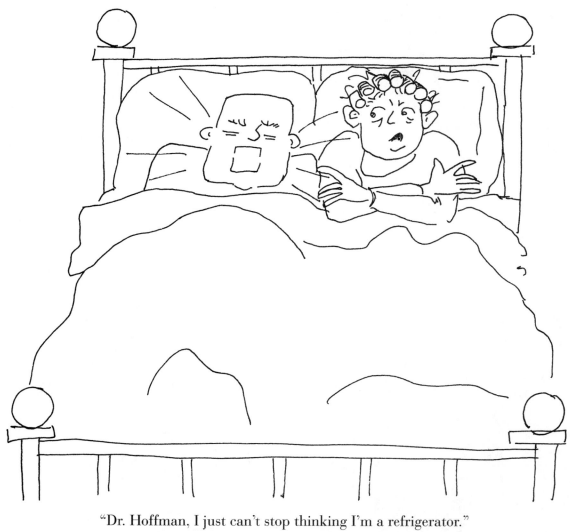

"Dr. Hoffman, I just can't stop thinking I'm a refrigerator."

"I see," said the doctor. "Does this disturb you?"

"Well, not really—"

"Well, then I wouldn't worry about it."

"Dr. Hoffman, I sleep with my mouth open."

"So?"

"The light keeps my wife awake all night long."

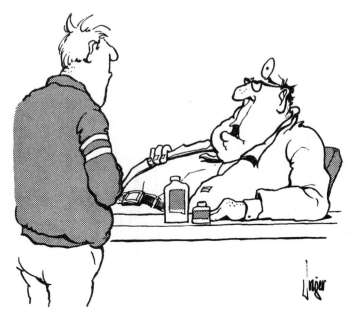

"Are you eating properly and getting plenty of exercise?"

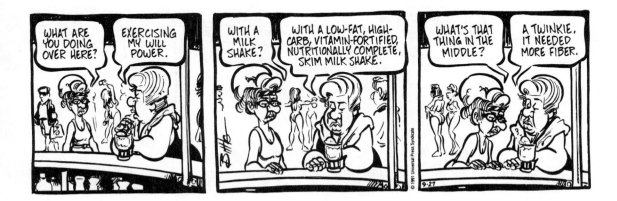

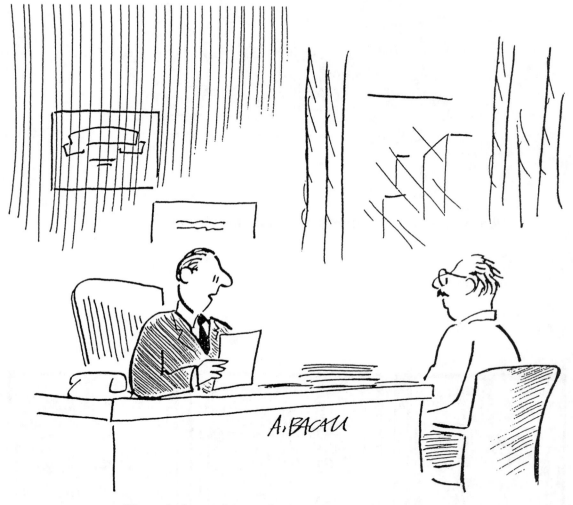

"Your cholesterol is too high and your fibre is too low.
Stop eating all those eggs and start eating the carton they come in."

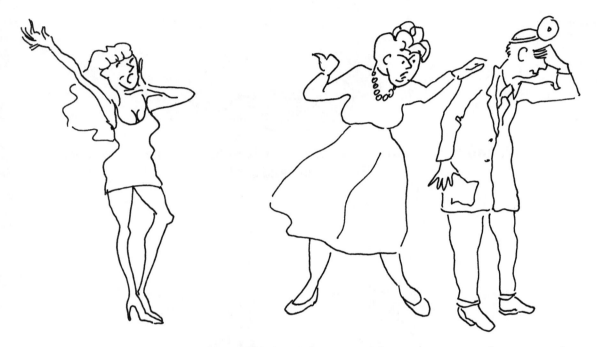

Dr. Morgan and his wife were walking down the street when a very attractive woman in a short skirt gave a little wave to the doctor.

"Who was that?" Mrs. Morgan inquired.

"Oh, just someone I know professionally," said the doctor.

"Oh, I see," Mrs. Morgan said. "Your profession, or hers?"

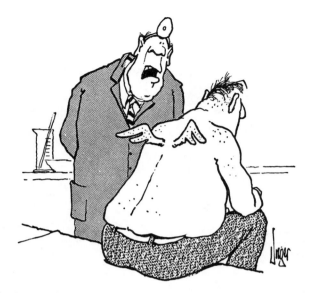

"Chicken for breakfast, chicken for lunch, chicken for dinner. What d'you expect?"

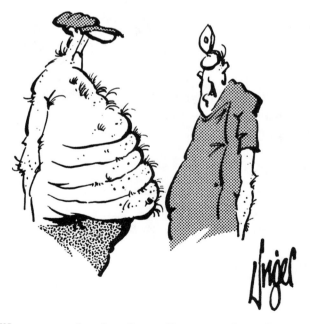

"I see you're back to five meals a day."

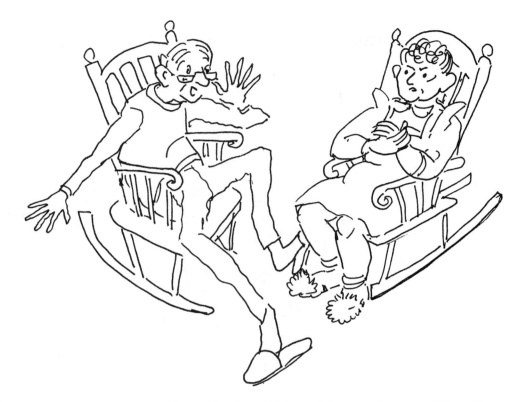

An elderly couple were celebrating their 50th wedding anniversary. The wife was eighty-two-years of age and her husband was eighty-six. It was a beautiful night, a full moon was coming up over the foothills, and they had cracked open a bottle of champagne at midnight.

They were both rocking comfortably, reminiscing about their life together, when suddenly the woman stood up from her rocking chair and walked over to her husband. For no apparent reason, she walked squarely up to his chair, faced him, and with no warning whatsoever, gave him a powerful whack across the face with her hand.

The husband, stunned, said, "What in the world did you do that for?"

"That was for fifty years of **bad** sex!" said the woman, as she returned to her chair.

Startled, the husband continued to rock in his chair. His face became increasingly flushed—livid with anger in fact—as thoughts churned through his mind. So without warning, he then stood up, walked over to his wife's chair, and gave her one powerful whack across her face with his hand.

"What did you do that for?"

"That," he said, "was for knowing the difference!"

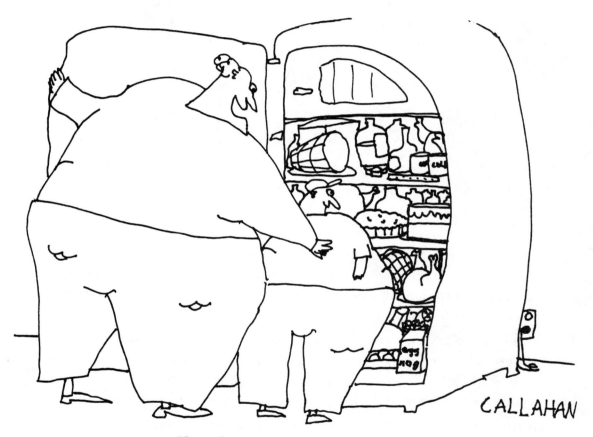

"Someday, son, all this will be yours!"

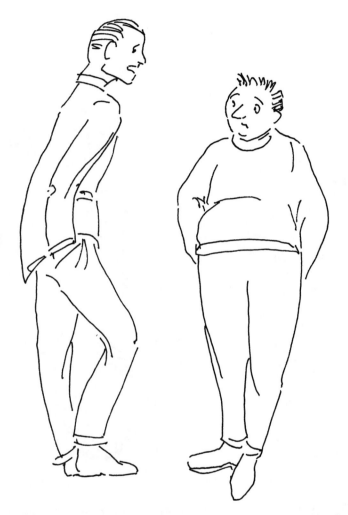

A man who had just been to his physician confided to his friend,
"My doctor said that if I didn't stop chasing women,
  I'd be dead before very long."

"That's a very strange thing for him to say," said his friend.

"Not really," the man said. "One of the women is his wife."

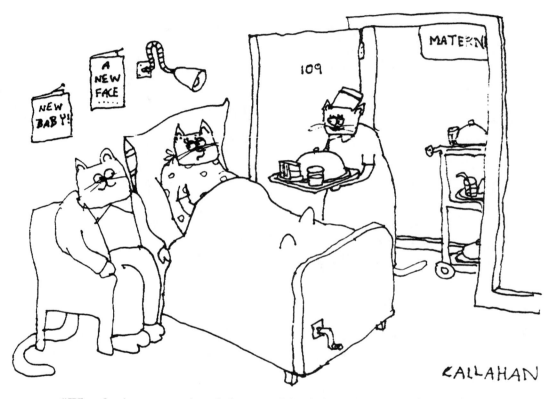

"Why don't you go ahead, honey—I had that placenta this morning."

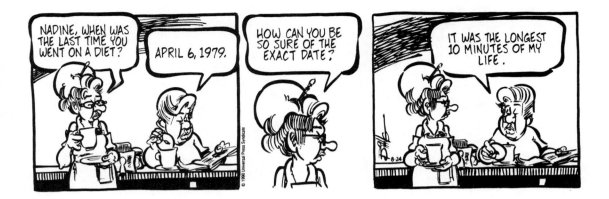

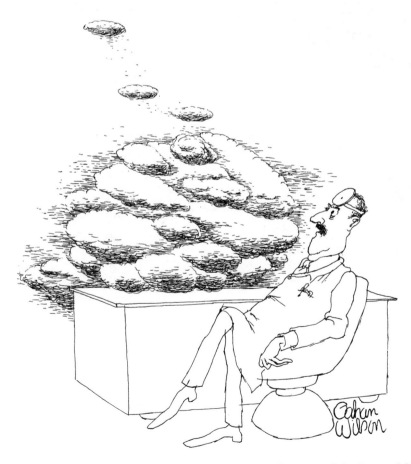

"How many cigarettes a day have you got it down to, Mr. Leopold?"

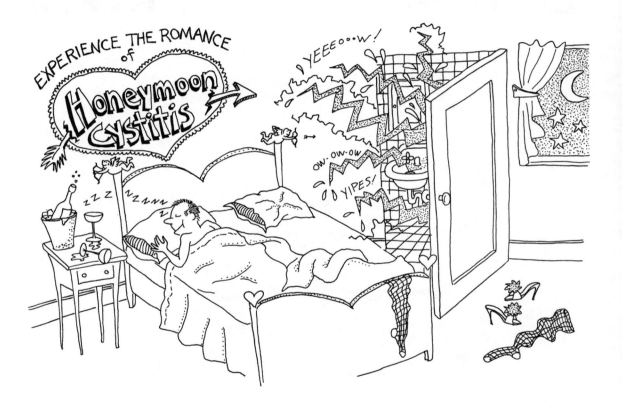

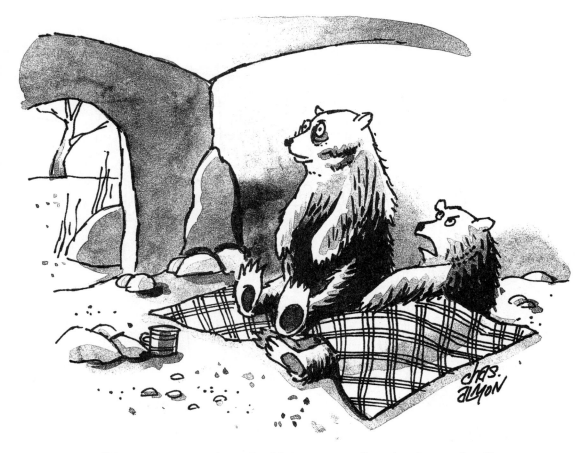

"How many times have I told you—no coffee after September!"

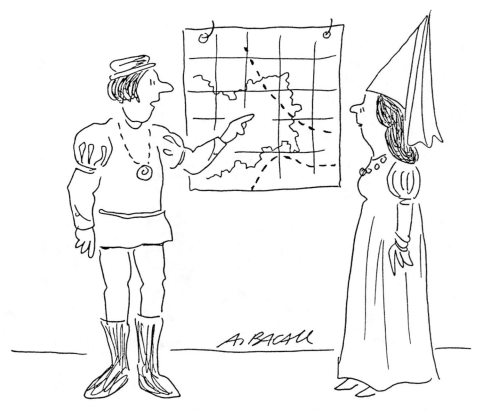

"What I propose to do, Isabella, is to take three ships on an easterly route in search of a salt substitute."

Nursing Your Wounds

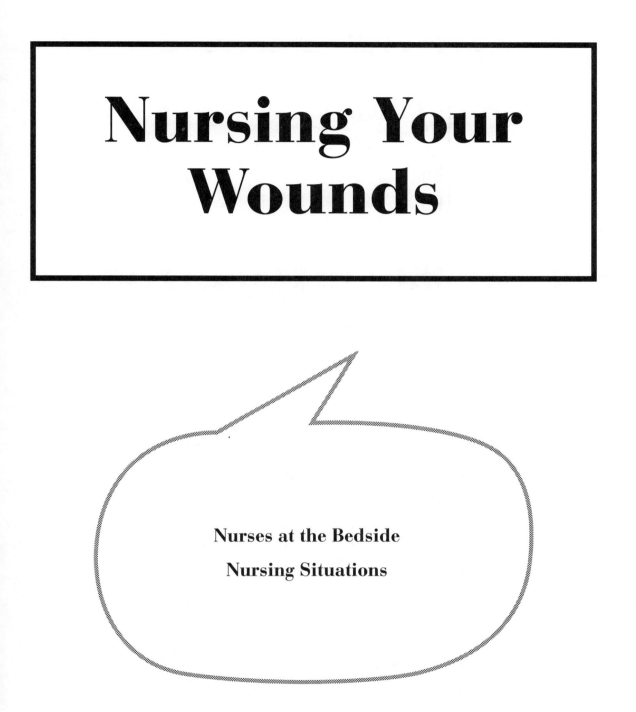

Nurses at the Bedside

Nursing Situations

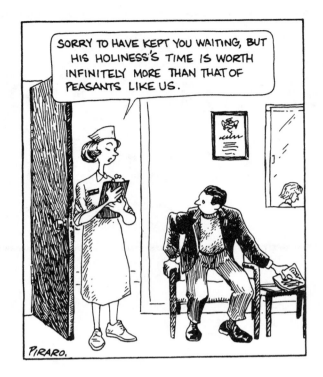

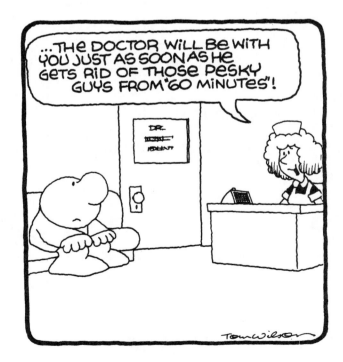

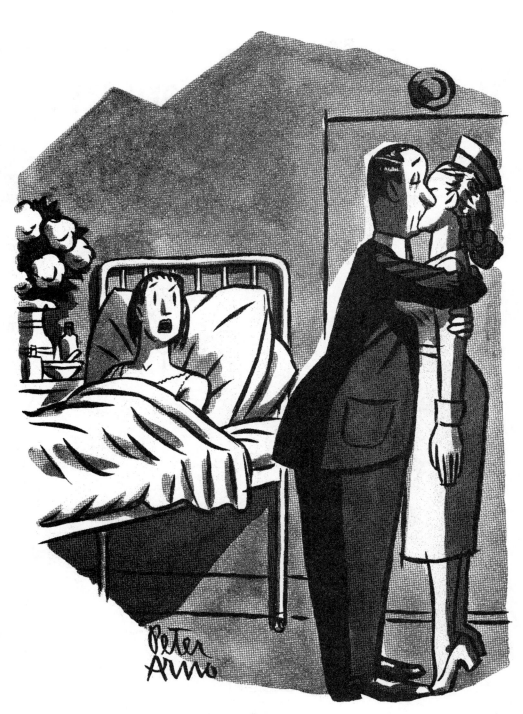

"George! It was **Dr. Carter** that pulled me through!"

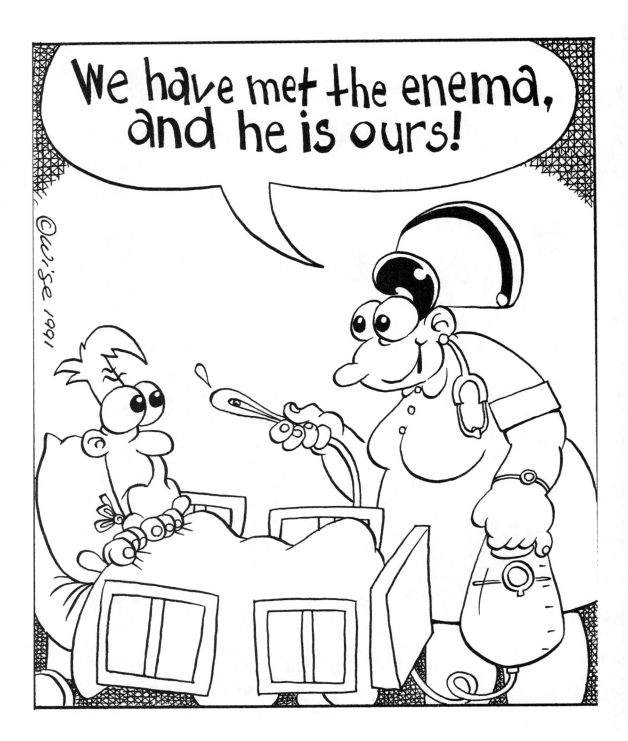

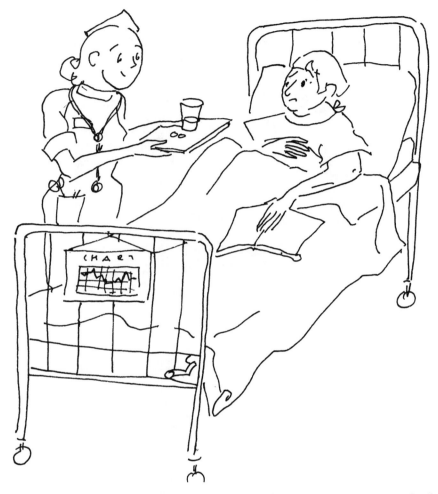

When the ward nurse came to give Mrs. Albrich her medicine, the patient looked askance at the pills.

"Excuse me," the patient said. "I was reading in a magazine about a woman who checked into this hospital because she had heart trouble—like me—and ended up dying because a nurse gave her the wrong medicine!"

The nurse just smiled.

"You can relax," Mrs. Albrich. "Rest assured, when people come into this hospital with heart trouble, they die **of heart trouble!**"

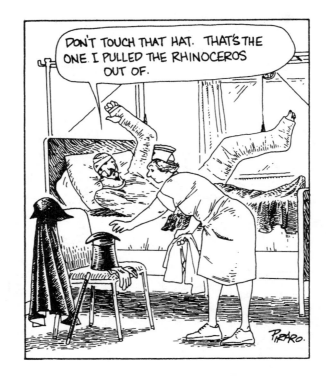

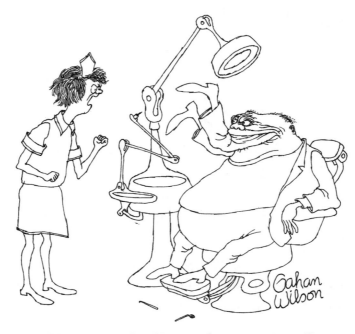

"You spit out Dr. Harper this very minute!"

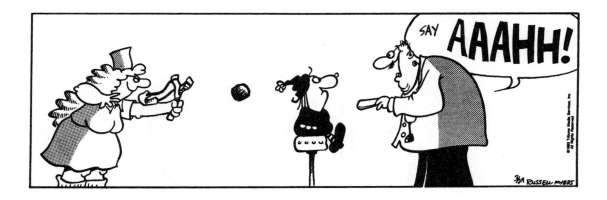

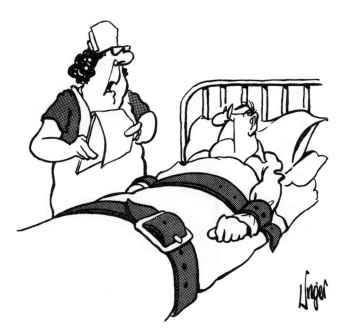

"Hospital regulations. You gotta wear the straps while I read the bill."

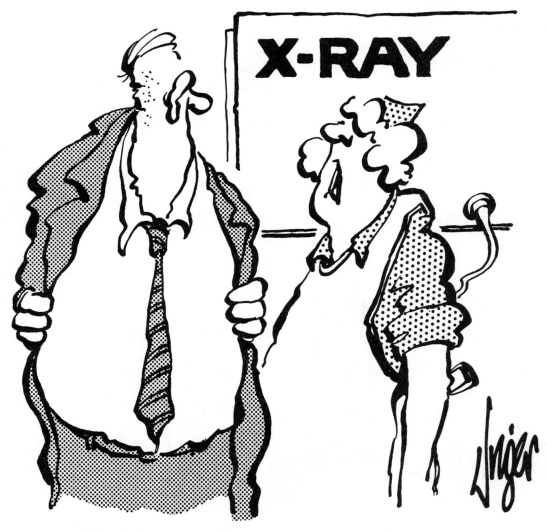

"Don't bother undressing. I'll turn up the power."

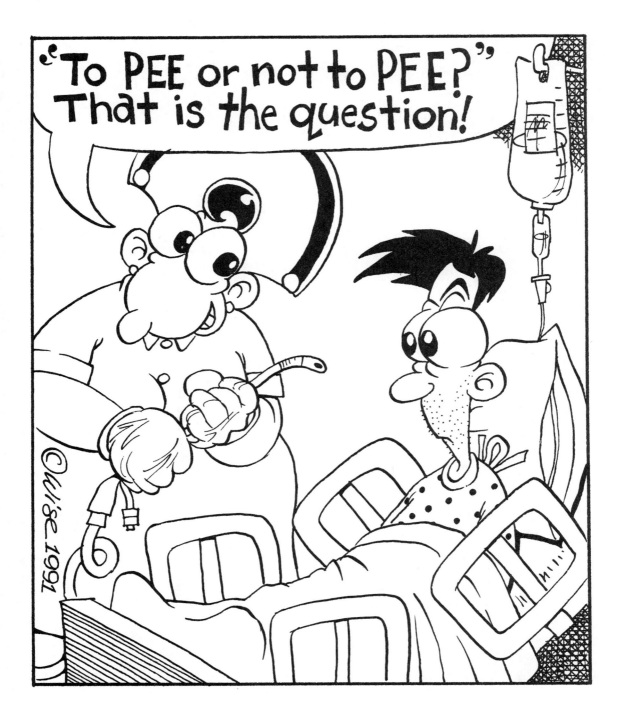

137

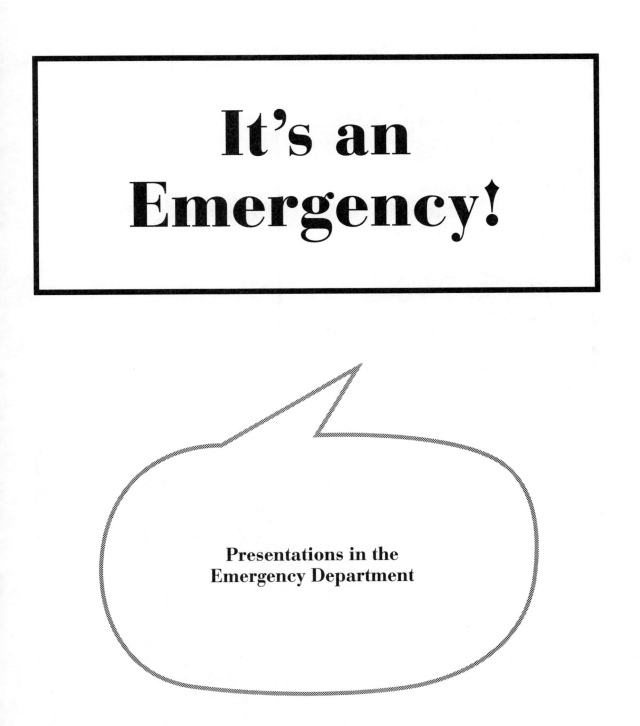

It's an Emergency!

Presentations in the
Emergency Department

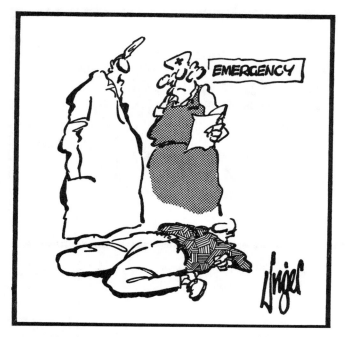

"Is this the 54-year-old limbo dancer?"

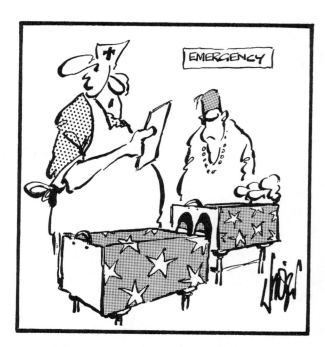

"Are you three all together?"

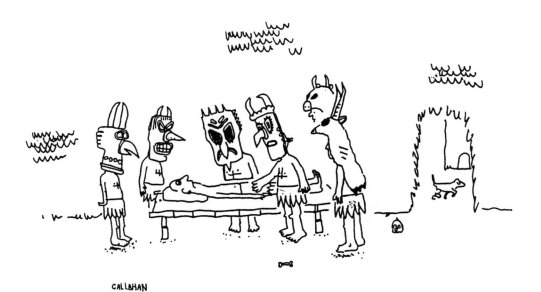

CALLAHAN

"This is a twenty-four-year-old male who was admitted last night with fever, chilling, and severe abdominal cramping. . . ."

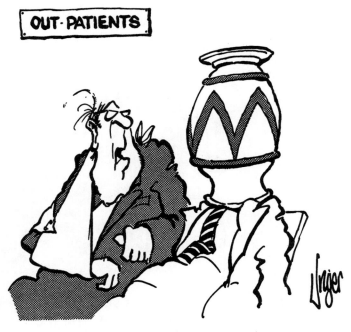

"What are you here for?"

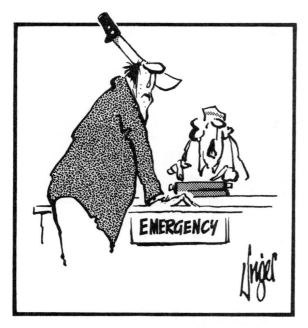

"Joyce, how do you spell 'juggling'?"

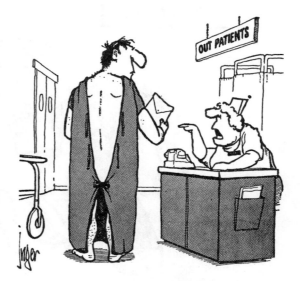

**"You go across the square, pass the nurse's residence,
up the steps, through the main lobby . . .
and second door on your left."**

The Chronologically Gifted

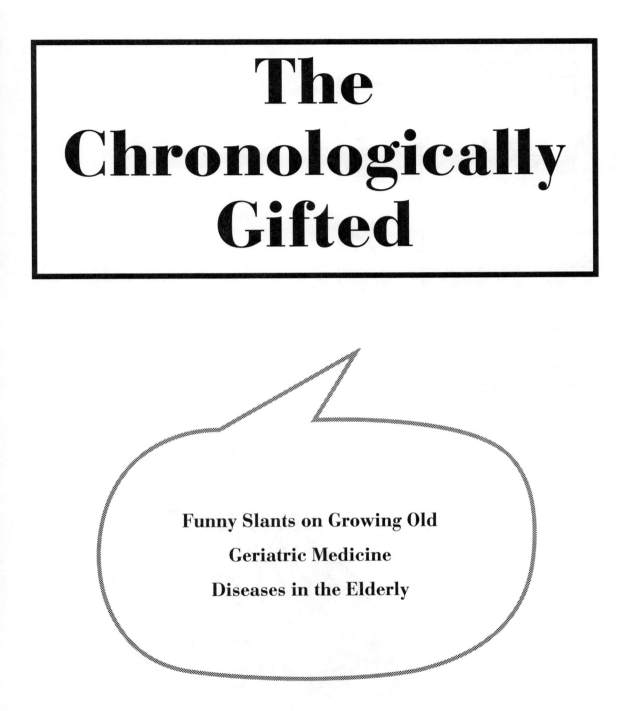

Funny Slants on Growing Old

Geriatric Medicine

Diseases in the Elderly

CLOSE TO HOME JOHN McPHERSON

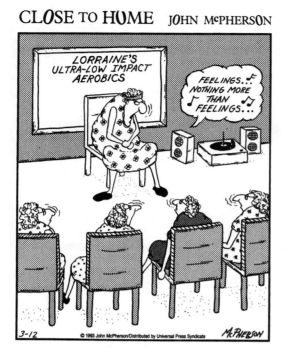

"OK, now the left nostril. Good!"

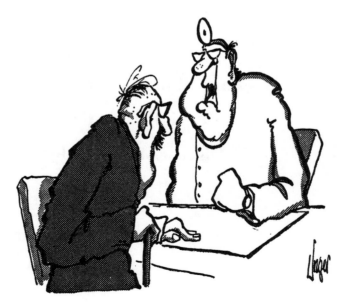

"I'm well aware you're only 28 years old.
That's why I'm telling you to take better care of yourself."

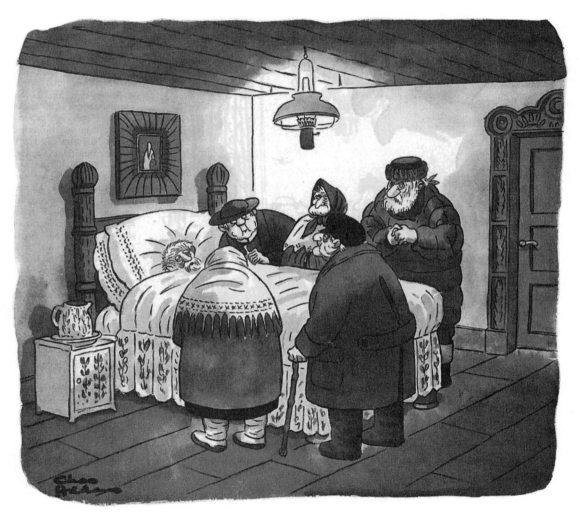

"To . . . hell . . . with . . . yogurt."

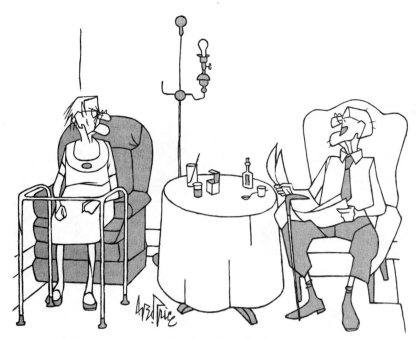

"Libra (September 23-October 23): Busy, busy, busy.
The accent is on excitement and romance.
Be ready for a flurry of calls, invitations . . ."

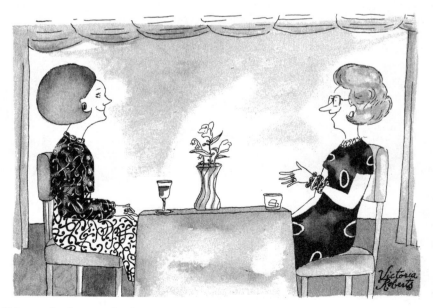

"Not only do you look marvelous, but all of you looks the same age."

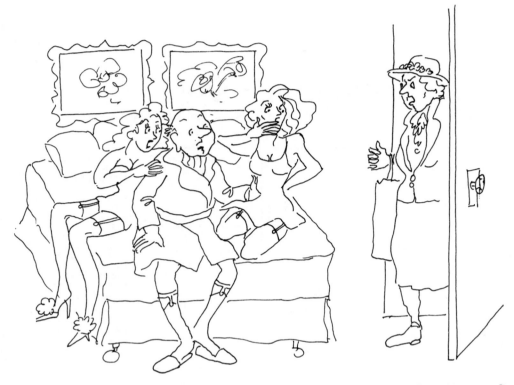

An elderly couple lived on the fourteenth floor of a very exclusive condominium in San Diego, California. One day, the woman went out shopping, as was her usual routine. She returned in the early afternoon after having lunch with her friends, and found her eighty-four-year-old husband in bed, under the sheets, with **two** twenty-five-year-old young ladies.

Unable to believe the sight before her eyes, the woman marched, as if in a trance, directly to the bed. Without hesitation, she ripped off the covers, picked her husband up by the scruff of the neck, marched him to the window, and **threw** him down fourteen floors to his death.

She returned back to the bed where the two young intruders had watched in horror.

"My God, why did you do that?" screamed one of the young women.

"If he can be in bed with you two young things," said the elderly woman, "he can fly!"

LIFE IN HELL

© 1989 BY MATT GROENING

HOW LONG WILL YOU LIVE?

A FUN TEST

START THIS FUN TEST WITH 73 LUCKY BONUS POINTS.

IF YOU ARE FEMALE, ADD 4.

IF MALE, SUBTRACT 5.

IF YOU LIVE ON A SMALL ISLAND IN THE SOUTH PACIFIC ALL BY YOURSELF, ADD 3.

IF YOU LIVE IN A SMALL APARTMENT IN A LARGE CITY WITH A ROOMMATE WHO WHISTLES, SUBTRACT 4.

IF ANY GRANDPARENT LIVED TO BE 93, ADD 2.

IF YOU HAD TO ATTEND ANY GRANDPARENT'S OPEN-CASKET FUNERAL, SUBTRACT 2.

IF YOU WORK BEHIND A DESK, SUBTRACT 2.

IF YOUR WORK REQUIRES LIFTING DESKS, SUBTRACT 3.

IF YOU WORK WITH COMPUTERS, SUBTRACT 2.

IF YOU DREAM ABOUT COMPUTERS, SUBTRACT 3.

IF YOU WORK ON A CATWALK ABOVE HUGE VATS OF NOXIOUS BOILING LIQUIDS, SUBTRACT 5.

IF YOU DRINK COFFEE, SUBTRACT 1.

DECAF IS HELL

IF YOU ARE ANNOYED BY THE PHRASE "HAVE A NICE DAY," SUBTRACT 3.

IF YOU HAVE EATEN A DONUT IN THE LAST 10 YEARS, SUBTRACT 4.

IF YOU HAVE EVER EVEN THOUGHT ABOUT GOING TO GRADUATE SCHOOL, SUBTRACT 2.

IF YOU GET INTO LOUD ARGUMENTS WITH STRANGERS ON BUSES, SUBTRACT 2.

I'M NO

IF YOU LIVE WITH A SPOUSE OR FRIEND, ADD 2.

IF THE SPOUSE OR FRIEND IS A POET, SUBTRACT 3.

IF YOU HAVE EVER WORN LEATHER PANTS, SUBTRACT 2.

IF YOU HAVE EVER DATED SOMEONE WHO WORE LEATHER PANTS, SUBTRACT 1.

YOO HOO.

IF YOU WEAR SUNGLASSES AT NIGHT, SUBTRACT 3.

IF YOU ARE IMPRESSED BY ROCK STARS WHO POUT, SUBTRACT 2.

IF YOU ARE IMPRESSED BY PERFORMANCE ARTISTS WHO PELT YOU WITH MEAT BY-PRODUCTS, SUBTRACT 3.

ARE YOU ANGRY AND VINDICTIVE, OR FROM NEW YORK? SUBTRACT 2.

ARE YOU RELAXED AND MELLOW? SUBTRACT 2.

ARE YOU HIP AND SELF-SATISFIED, OR FROM LOS ANGELES? SUBTRACT 3.

IF YOU RESENT THIS TEST, SUBTRACT 3.

VOILÀ!!

YOUR SCORE AT THIS POINT IS YOUR LIFE EXPECTANCY.

Have a nice day.

10·27·1989 ACME FEATURES SYNDICATE © 1989 BY MATT GROENING

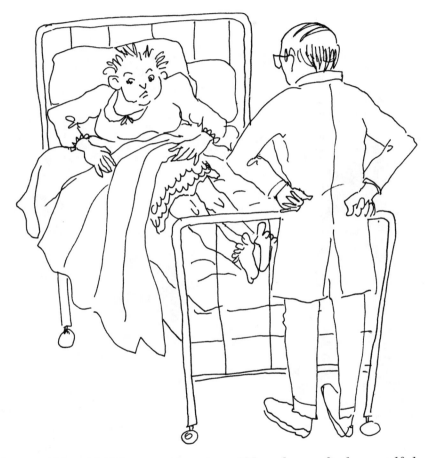

"So," the doctor said to his 87-year-old patient, "How do you find yourself these days?"

"As I always have," said the woman. "I just throw back the covers each morning and there I am!"

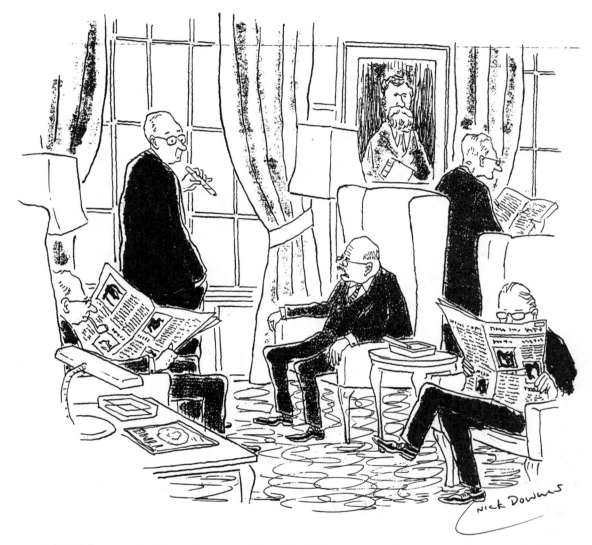

"*Would you mind stepping out of the light? I've got a solar-powered pacemaker.*"

150

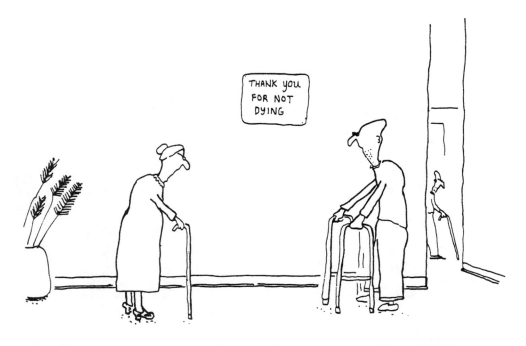

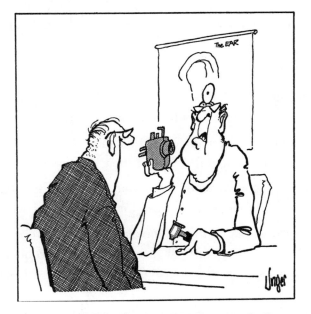

"We implant this behind your left ear
and you won't even know it's there."

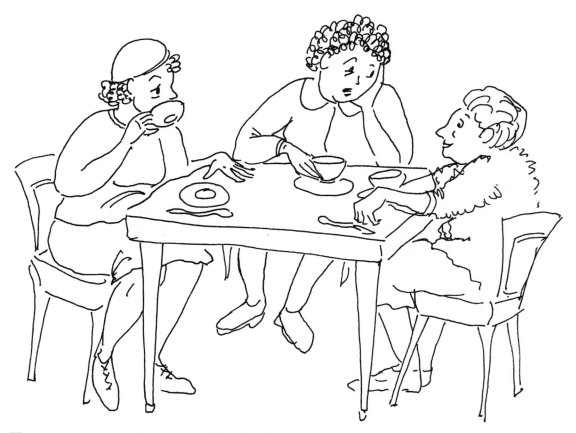

Three women were sitting around at lunch one day talking about the memory difficulties that they were beginning to experience with the march of time.

One woman said, "You know, it's terrible. I go to a show, I recognize the movie stars, but by the time I get home, I can't remember any of their names."

The second woman said, "I know exactly what you mean. I go to a restaurant and place an order and by the time the food arrives, I can't even remember what I ordered."

"Not me," offered the third woman. "I don't have any of those problems. "In fact," she said adamantly, knocking her hand against the surface of the wooden table, "My memory is every bit as good today as it was thirty years ago . . . by the way, who's knocking at the door?"

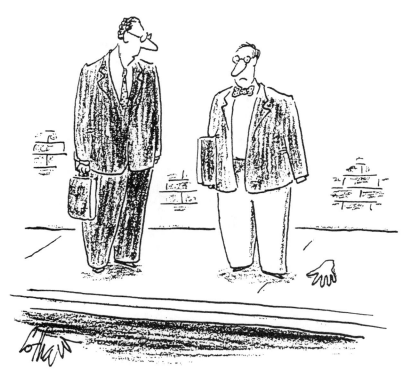

"Nothing to worry about, it's all part of the aging process."

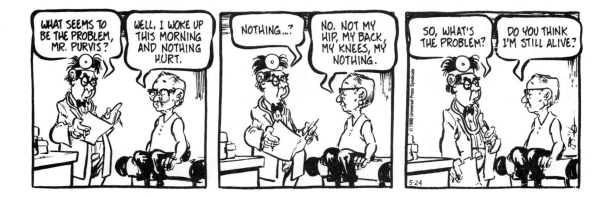

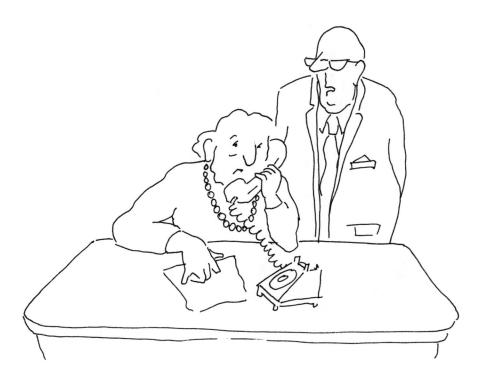

An eighty-six-year-old woman named Betty called her attorney. "Hello John, this is Betty," said the woman.

"Hello, Betty," said John. "What can I do for you?"

"Well," said Betty, "Fred and I have decided that we would like a divorce."

"A divorce?" said her lawyer, "A divorce, Betty? Now? Are you sure about this?"

"Yes, very sure," Betty said.

"I don't quite understand," her lawyer confided. "You're eighty-six-years-old. Fred is eighty-eight. And you want a divorce now?" "Why now?"

"Well," said Betty. "Fred and I talked it over, and we thought it would be nice to wait until the kids were dead."

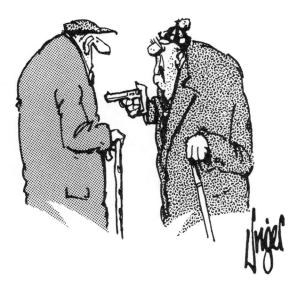

"Hand over your pacemaker."

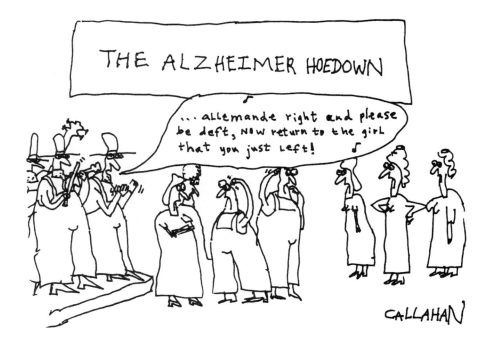

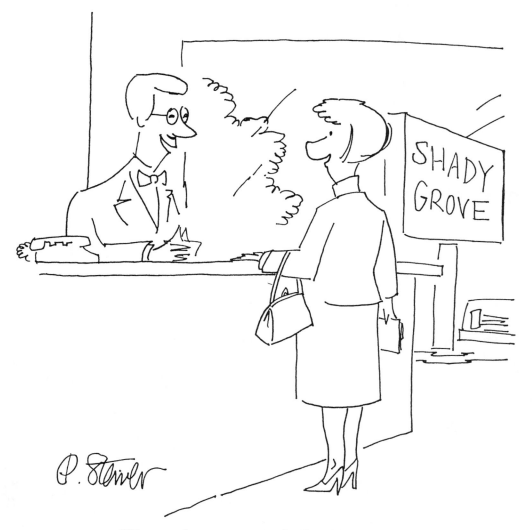

"*We are a long-term care facility, Mrs. Williams,*
which means that over the long term you will get some care."

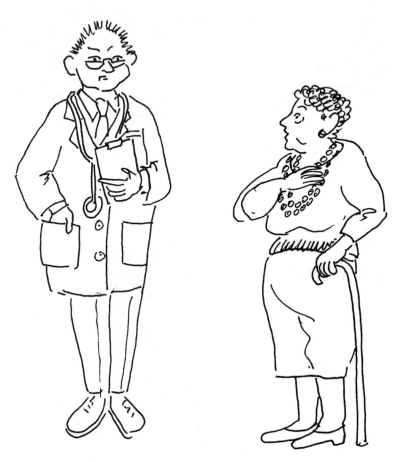

A very anxious elderly woman entered her doctor's office to receive results of tests that had been performed a few days ago.

"Well," said the doctor, "I have some good news and some bad news."

"Let's hear it," said the woman.

"The good news," the doctor said, "is that your HIV test is negative. And the bad news," he continued, "is that your CAT scan shows that you probably have Alzheimer's disease."

"What a relief," the woman said. "I'm just glad to know I don't have Alzheimer's disease."

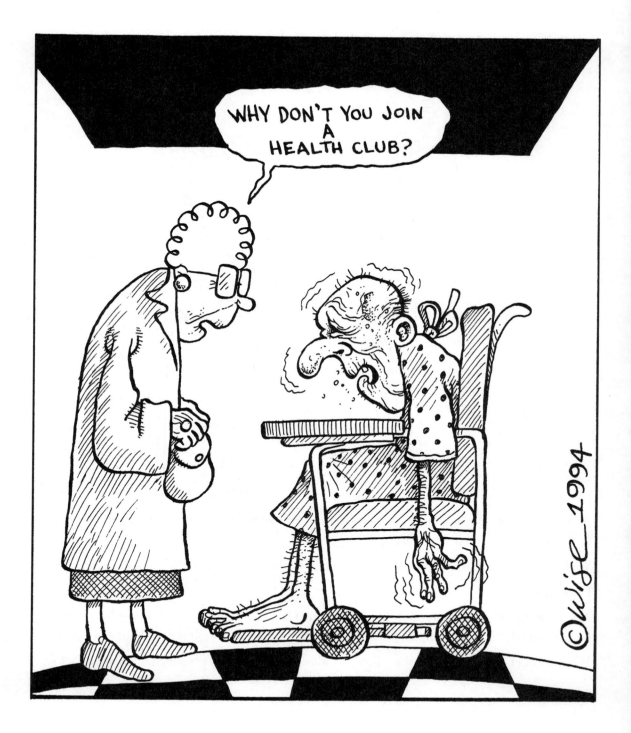

Funny Bones

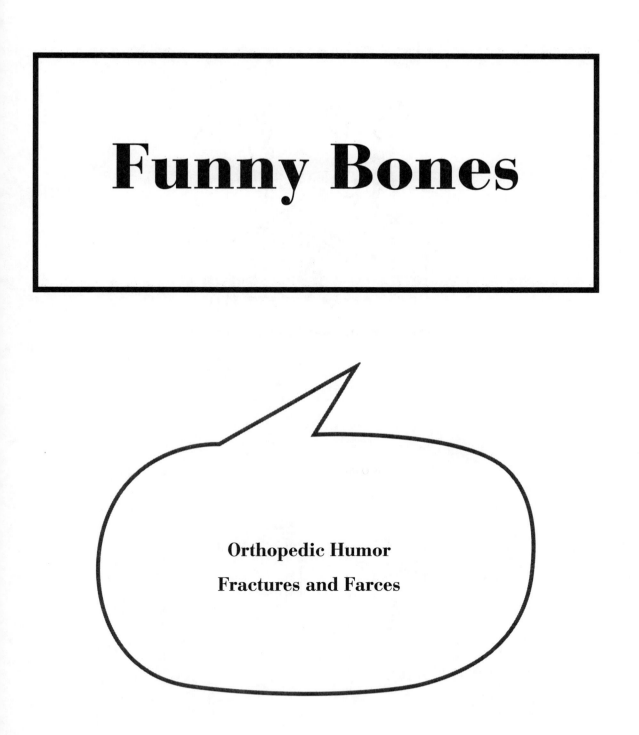

Orthopedic Humor

Fractures and Farces

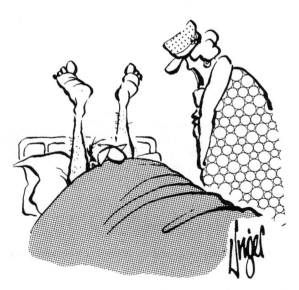

"They're gonna settle out of court."

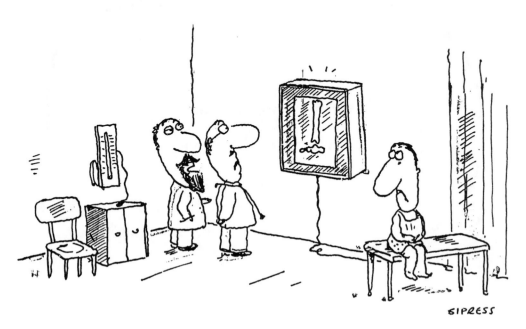

I like the feeling in this one, but I think you could have done more with the composition.

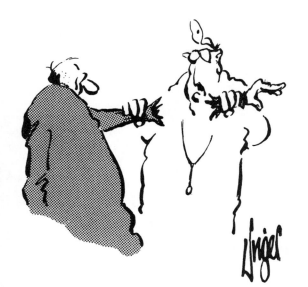

"Does that hurt?"

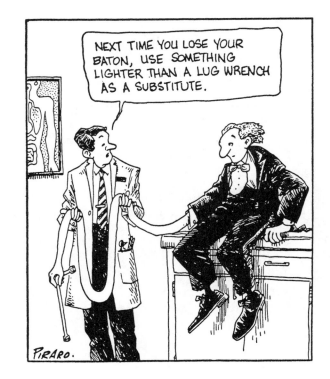

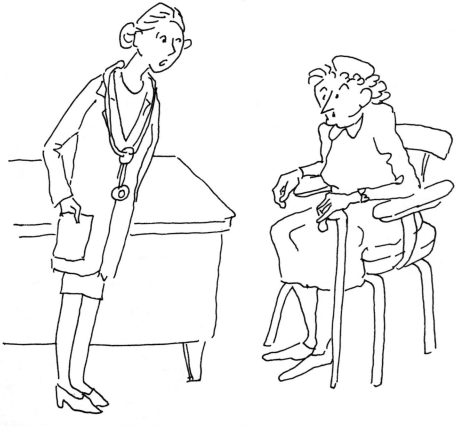

"Do you suffer from arthritis?" the doctor asked her patient.
"I sure do," the patient responded. "What else do you do with it?"

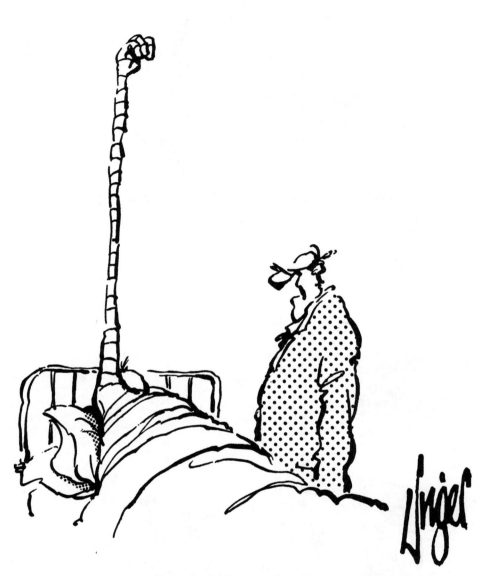

"Your wife says you stopped a runaway horse."

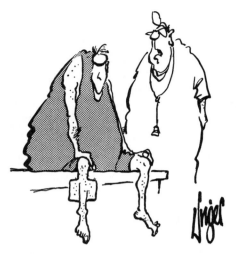

"We had to put a steel plate in your leg."

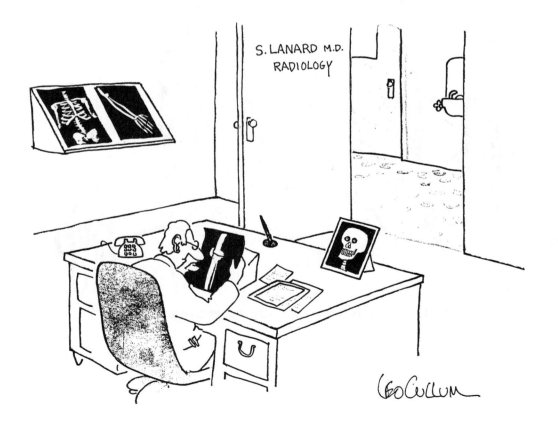

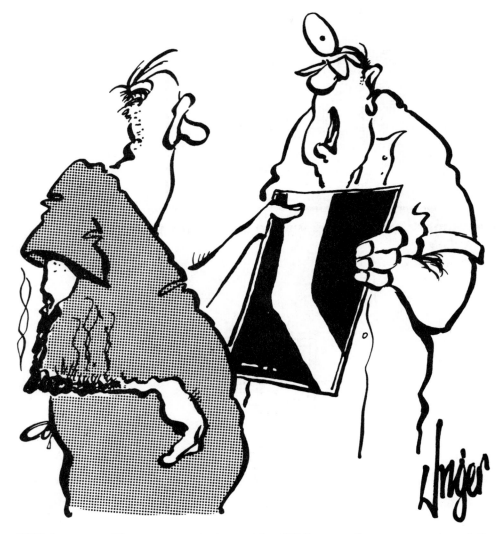

"I'll have to X-ray your arm again. This one is overexposed."

165

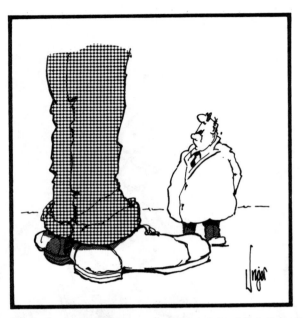

"As I remember, you always were a big kid for your age."

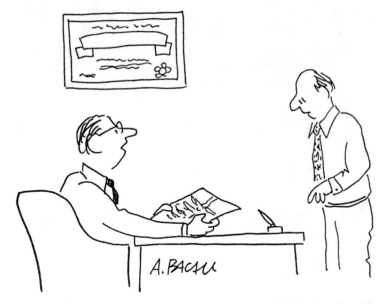

*"Tell your wife that the X-ray shows that you **do** have a backbone."*

The Grin Reaper

Death and Dying

Funeral Experiences

Humor in the Morgue

Suicide Made Light

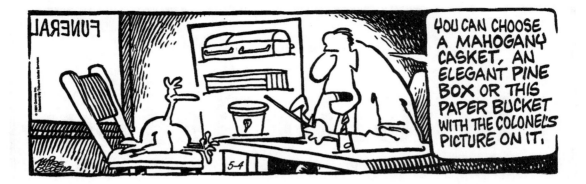

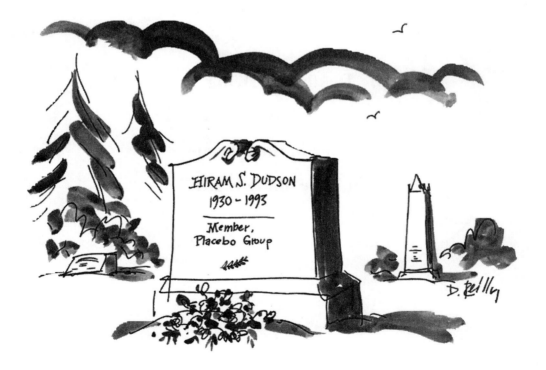

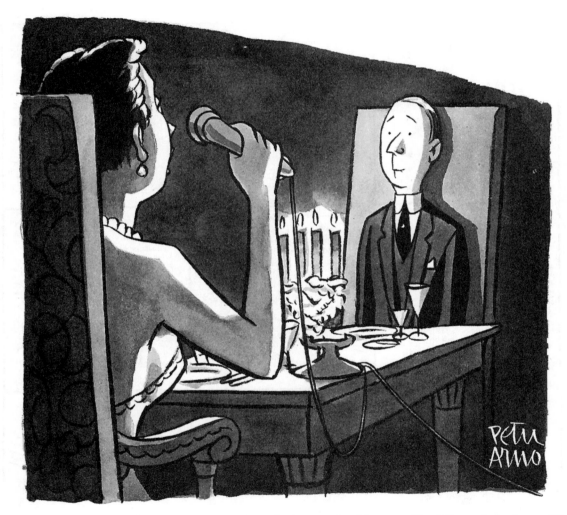

"There's someone who answers your description at the Morgue. Shall I say it isn't you?"

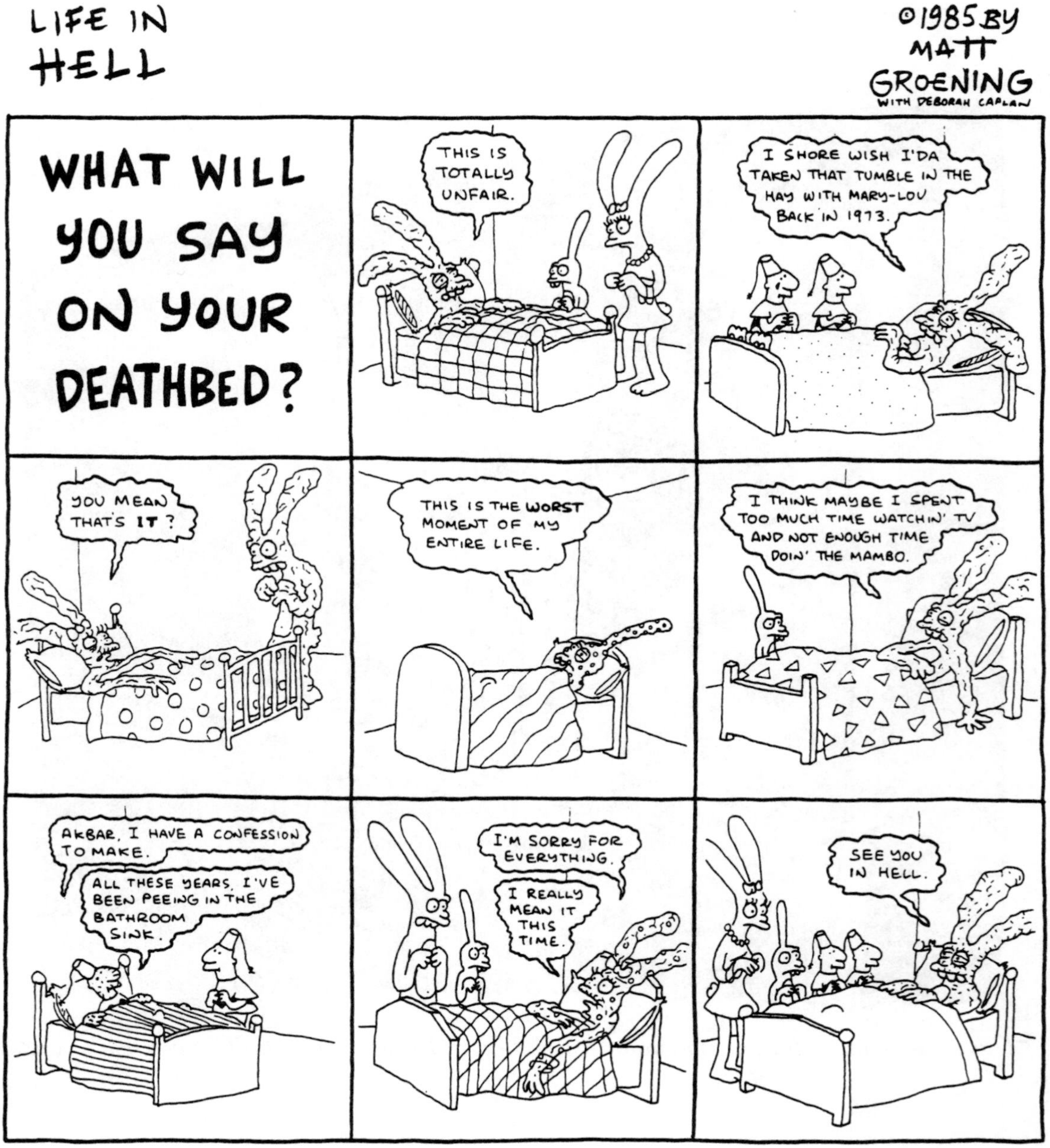
LIFE IN
HELL
©1985 BY
MATT
GROENING
WITH DEBORAH CAPLAN
WHAT WILL YOU SAY ON YOUR DEATHBED?
THIS IS TOTALLY UNFAIR.
I SHORE WISH I'DA TAKEN THAT TUMBLE IN THE HAY WITH MARY-LOU BACK IN 1973.
YOU MEAN THAT'S IT?
THIS IS THE WORST MOMENT OF MY ENTIRE LIFE.
I THINK MAYBE I SPENT TOO MUCH TIME WATCHIN' TV AND NOT ENOUGH TIME DOIN' THE MAMBO.
AKBAR, I HAVE A CONFESSION TO MAKE.
ALL THESE YEARS, I'VE BEEN PEEING IN THE BATHROOM SINK.
I'M SORRY FOR EVERYTHING.
I REALLY MEAN IT THIS TIME.
SEE YOU IN HELL.

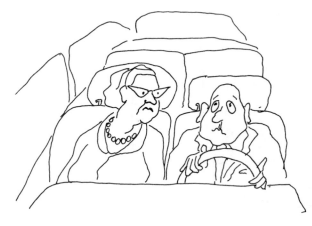

An elderly retired couple were very very active. However, the husband, Bill Morgan, however, suffered a heart attack at the age of sixty-nine. His wife was very concerned about his illness and, during his recovery period, decided that she would take all the precautions that she could to prolong his life. So she loaded Bill into their RV and drove all the way from Portland, Oregon to Rochester, Minnesota so that her husband could benefit from one of those comprehensive, mega-cardiac evaluations for which the Mayo Clinic is so famous. The husband sailed through all the diagnostic evaluations.

After completing the work-up, the husband—along with his wife—returned to the cardiologist's office for their final consultation and exit interview. The cardiologist looked at the man and said, "Bill, would you mind stepping out of the room for a few minutes? I would like to have a private conversation with your wife." The husband left the room.

"Well doctor," she inquired of the doctor, "Is there **anything** I can do to improve my husband's condition . . . you know—to prolong his life?"

"Absolutely," said the cardiologist, "I am sure you know that diet is very important for patients who have had a heart attack. Stated simply, your husband needs to be on three square, low-fat, low-cholesterol meals a day."

"No problem," said the woman. "Can I do anything else?"

"Yes," said the cardiologist, "Patients who have had a heart attack also need emotional support, love, and intimacy. In this regard, I believe your husband needs to have sex **every night**."

The woman thought about this for a moment and scribbled the cardiologist's recommendations down on a piece of paper to remind herself. Then she said, "Now, let me see if I have this straight. If I provide my husband three square, low-fat, low-cholesterol meals every day and sex every night, do you guarantee to me that his prognosis will be improved and that his life will be prolonged?"

"You have my word," said the doctor.

So the woman and her husband got back into their RV and started heading back to Portland. On the journey home, the husband turned to his wife and said, "Dear, is there anything else I should know about my condition?"

"Yep," she said, "You're going to **die, Bill!**"

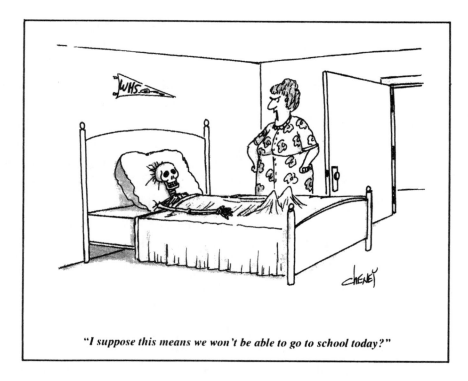

"I suppose this means we won't be able to go to school today?"

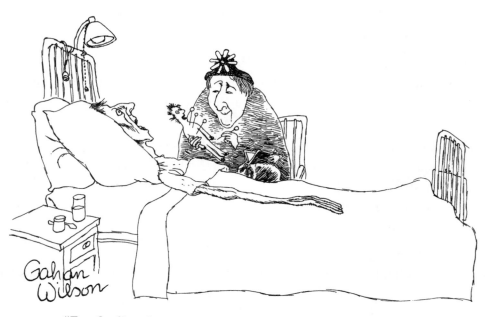

"For God's sake, Leona, why don't you just finish me off?"

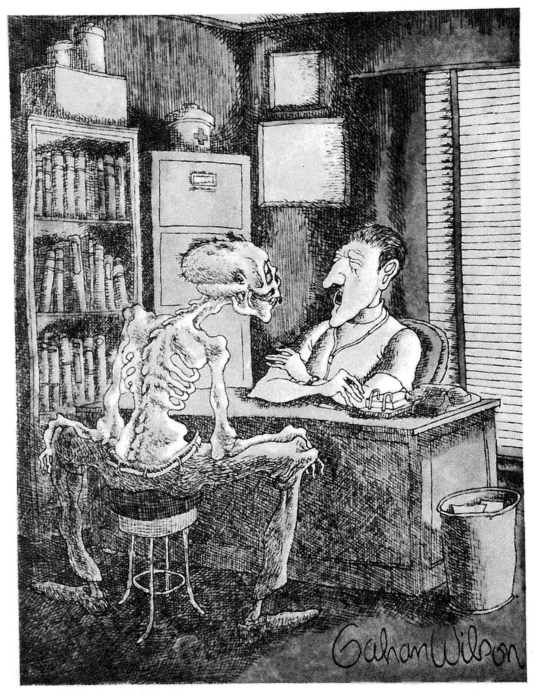

"We may already be too late, Mr. Parker."

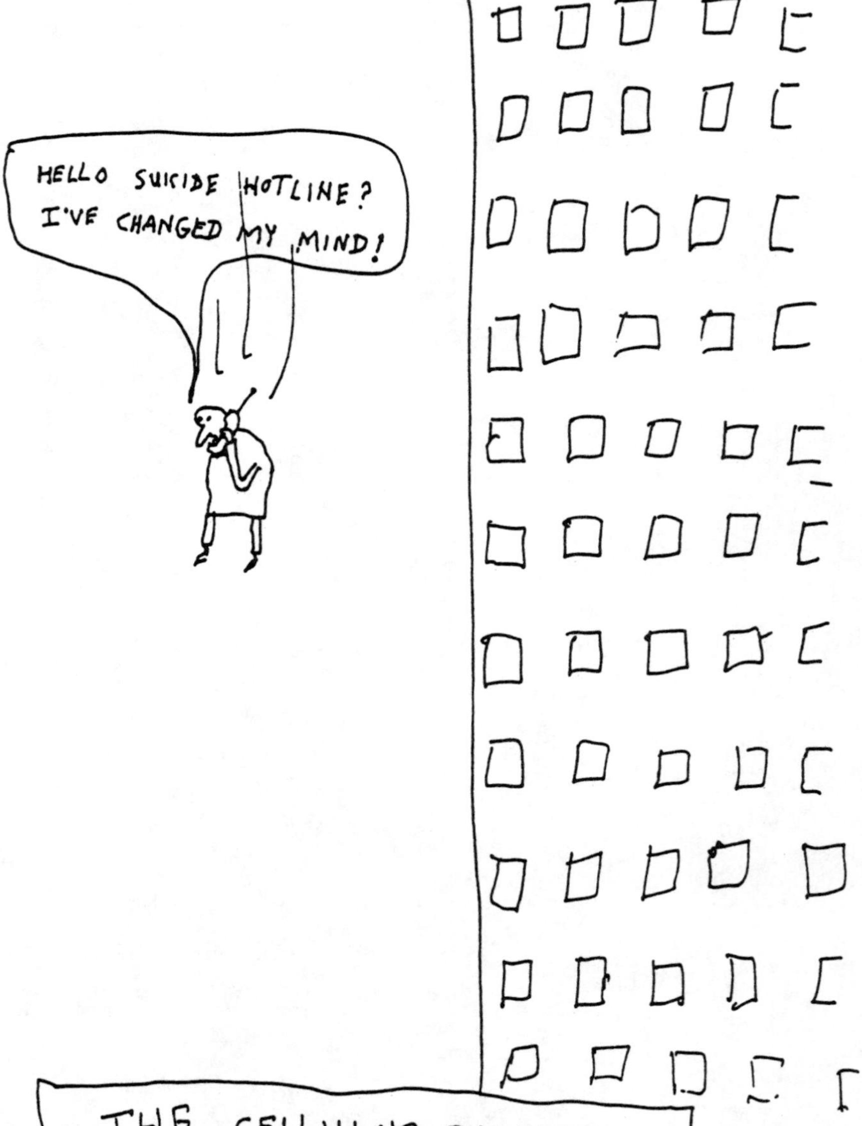
HELLO SUICIDE HOTLINE?
I'VE CHANGED MY MIND!
THE CELLULAR PHONE
CALLAHAN

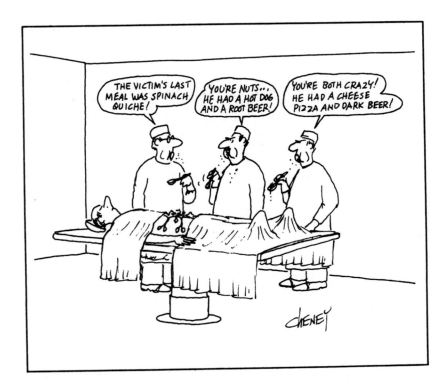

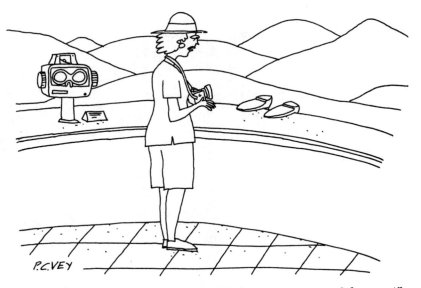

"Stop it! You know the doctor said that was no good for you!"

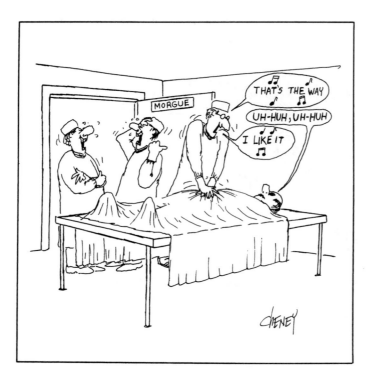

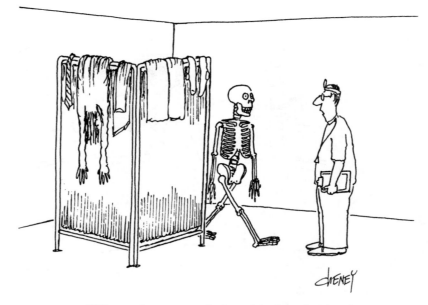

"Uh . . . just your clothes, Mr. Maybridge."

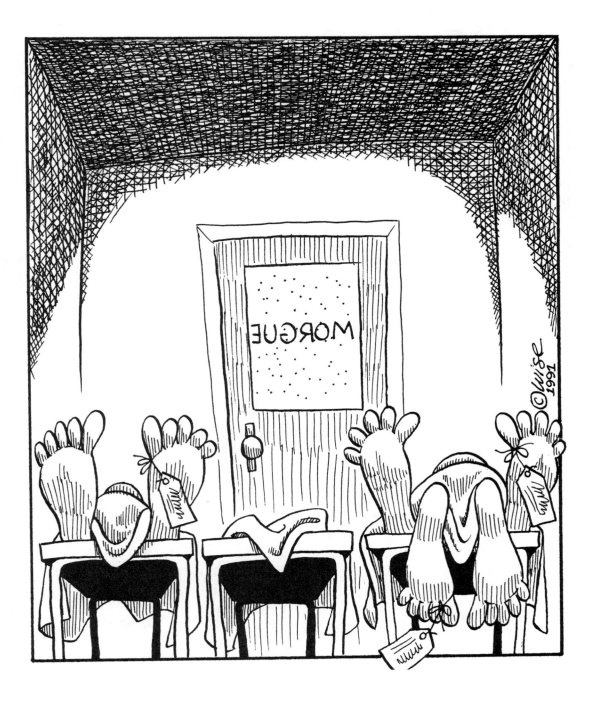

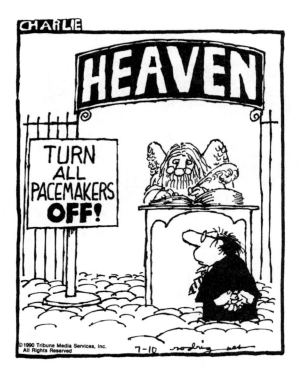

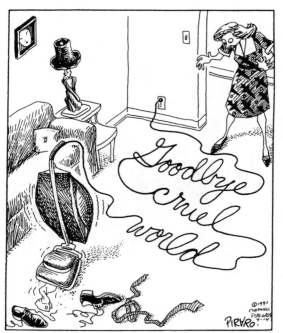

BIZARRO   By DAN PIRARO

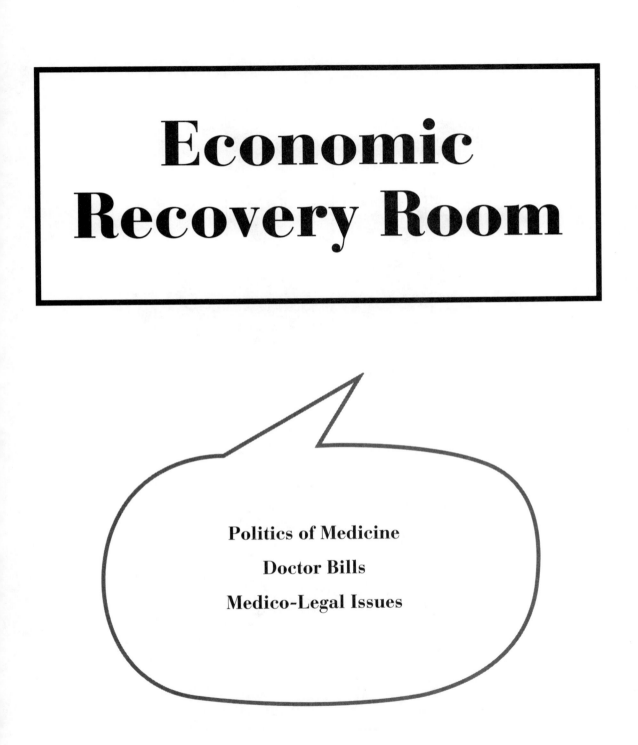

Economic Recovery Room

Politics of Medicine

Doctor Bills

Medico-Legal Issues

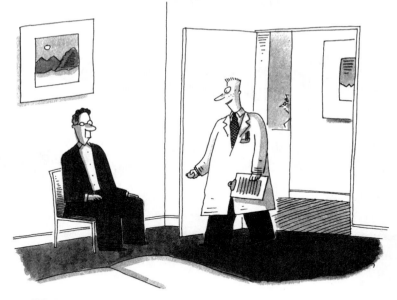

"Hi! My name is Kevin, and I'll be your doctor today."

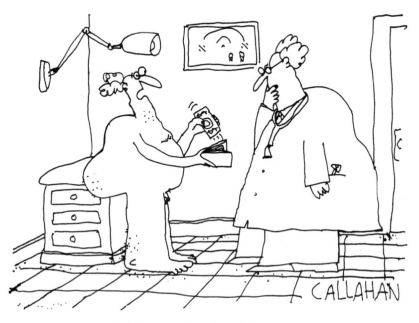

"It hurts when I go like this!"

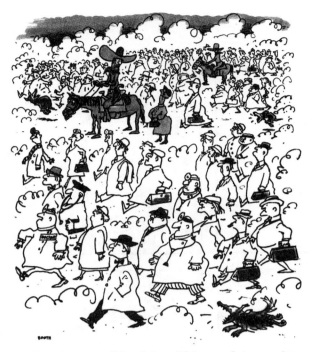

"The Discount Physicians' Network is moving two thousand head up to Dodge City, Ma'am."

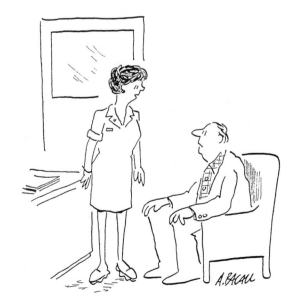

"The doctor will see your medical insurance coverage now."

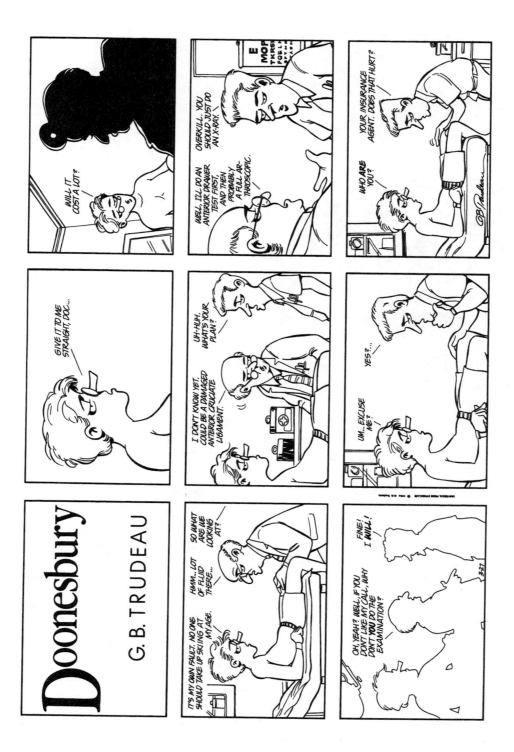

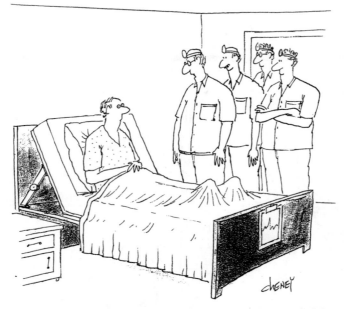

*"Bob, these are doctors Burton, Kane, and Rotlefield . . .
they'll be assisting me with your health insurance forms."*

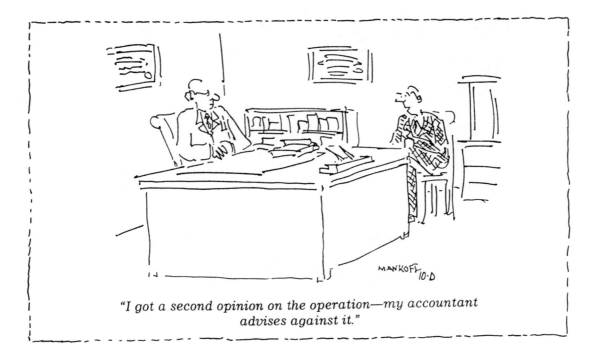

*"I got a second opinion on the operation—my accountant
advises against it."*

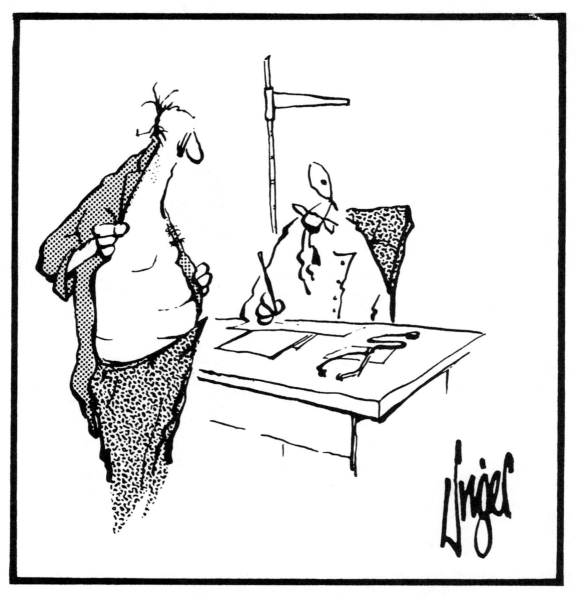

"Do you want to know what's wrong with you
or just the dollar amount?"

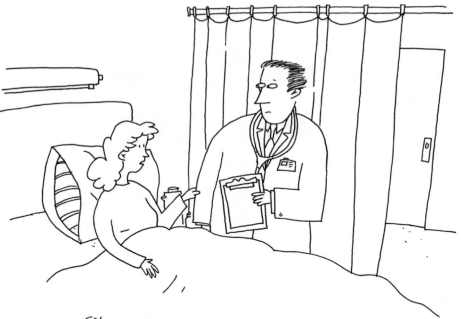

PCVEY

"I'm leaving you, John. My insurance ran out."

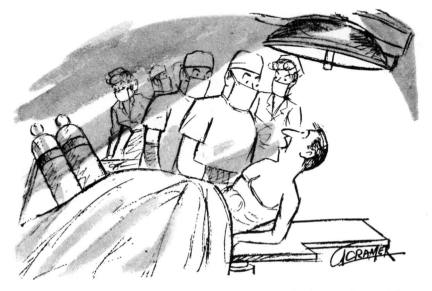

"Just one last thing . . . which credit cards do you honor?"

185

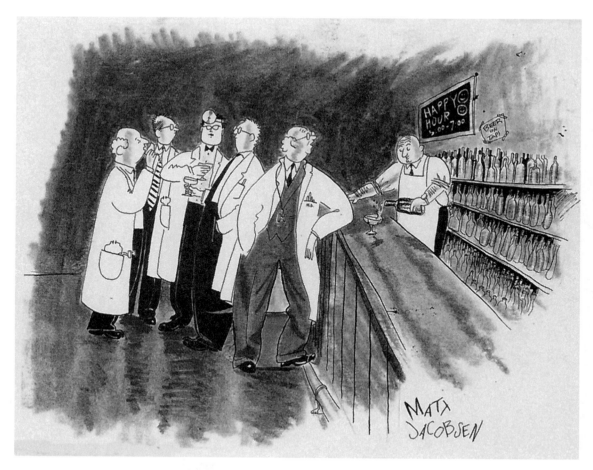

"If we should begin to toast the single-payer plan, cut us off."

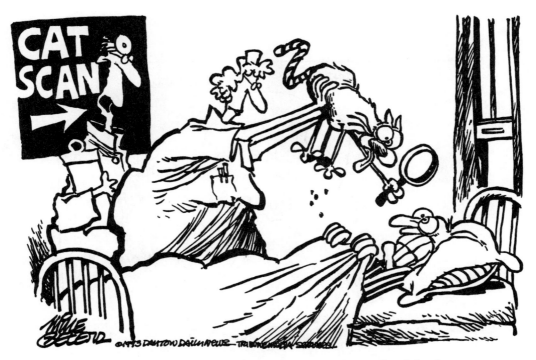

You have to expect some cutbacks with the Clinton health plan . . .

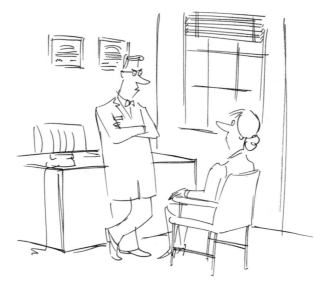

"If you want a second opinion, I'm sure Mrs. Clinton will be glad to oblige."

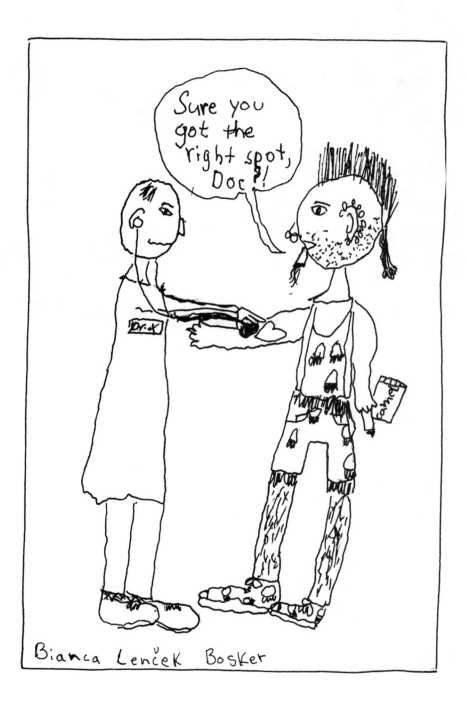

Credits